MINDFULNESS
FOR
CHALLENGING
TIMES

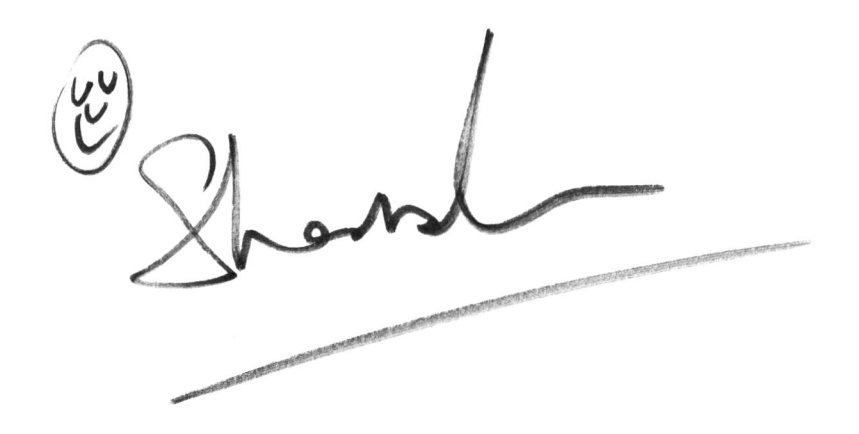

Testimonials

"Mindfulness is a vital skill to practise in our current highly challenging environment. This book is a wonderful gift to the world – a collaboration of voices to offer presence, compassion and hope, all for a good cause. I highly recommend!"

Shauna Shapiro PhD, author of *Good Morning, I Love You*
Professor, Santa Clara University

"Mindfulness seems so simple to do and yet so hard to describe. Shamash does it brilliantly."

Ruby Wax, comedian, mental health campaigner and bestselling author

"Shamash has a rare gift as a mindfulness teacher. A combination of clarity, compassion, authenticity and deep wisdom that makes you feel both warmly welcomed and confident you're in great hands. In this book, Shamash gives you the tools you need to guide you through challenging times and come out the other side stronger than you were before. It has his signature style of warmth, genuine care and crystal-clear practical tools. You couldn't find a better friend to guide you through troubled times."

Melli O'Brien, mindfulness teacher, speaker, writer and co-founder of Mindfulness.com

MINDFULNESS FOR CHALLENGING TIMES

A Collection of Voices for
Peace, Self-care and Connection

Notice of Liability: The author has made every effort to check and ensure the accuracy of the information presented in this book. However, the information herein is sold without warranty, either expressed or implied. Neither the author, publisher, nor any dealer or distributor of this book will be held liable for any damages caused either directly or indirectly by the instructions and information contained in this book.

Disclaimer: Information in this book is NOT intended as medical advice, or for use as diagnosis or treatment of a health problem, or as a substitute for consulting a licensed medical professional. The contents and information in this book are for informational use only and are not intended to be a substitute for professional medical advice, diagnosis or treatment. Always seek the advice of your physician or other qualified health provider for medical conditions. Never disregard professional medical advice or delay in seeking it because of something you read in this book.

Copyright © 2020 Shamash Alidina

All rights reserved. This book or any portion thereof may not be reproduced or used in any manner whatsoever without the express written permission of the author except for the use of brief quotations in a book review.

First printing, 2020

ShamashAlidina.com

TeachMindfulnessOnline.com

Cover Design: Emily Canino
Editors: Kerry Laundon and Rachael Chilvers

Table of Contents

Testimonials ii
Dedication xiii
Acknowledgements xiv
Foreword xv
The Story Behind This Book xvii
Introduction How to Use Mindfulness in Challenging Times
.... xix
    Inner Advisor Reflection xxii
    How to Use This Book xxii
    About Shamash Alidina xxiv

PART 1 MEETING CHALLENGES WITH MINDFULNESS 1

1 Finding Calm in the Chaos 3
    How Mindfulness Can Help 5
    A Little Neuroscience 6
    Changing Our Perception 7
    PACE: A Mindfulness Practice 7
    Remember: 10
    About Dawn Andrews 11

2 Staying Mindful in Isolation 13
    Connect 13
    Be Selective, Be a Detective 14
    Pay Attention to What You Can Control 15

Mindfulness in Motion 16
　　Remember: 17
　　About Terry McCoy 18
3 Finding Ways to Cope with Stress 19
　　Your Body's Response to Stress 20
　　What Are the Key Sources of Stress? 20
　　Healthy and Unhealthy Ways to Cope with Stress 22
　　Mindful Exercises to Help Ease Stress 22
　　Remember: 24
　　About Pierpaolo Paparo 26
4 Mindfulness for Anxiety 27
　　What is Anxiety? 28
　　How Does Mindfulness Help with Anxiety? 30
　　The Science Behind Dealing with Anxiety 31
　　Techniques for Soothing Anxious Thoughts 32
　　Remember: 34
　　About Caitriona Horan 35
5 Managing Sleep in Challenging Times 37
　　Understanding Your Sleep Cycle 38
　　The Stages of Sleep 39
　　My Sleep Story 39
　　Debunking Some Common Myths About Sleep 40
　　Tips for Sleeping Well During Difficult Times 43
　　Remember: 44
　　About Jane Bozier 46

6 Mindfulness in the Presence of Traumatic Memories 47

Fight/Flight/Freeze and the Post-traumatic Response 48

Mindfulness in Challenging Times, alongside Traumatic Memories 50

Modifications for Practising Mindfulness with Trauma 51

Grounding and Supportive Trauma-aware Meditations 53

Remember: 54

About Amy Malloy 56

7 Being Mindful with Grief 57

How Do We Deal with Grief Mindfully? 58

Using Self-care with Grief 59

Crafting a Programme of Self-care 60

Moving towards Acceptance 62

Remember: 63

About Linda Shalloe 64

8 A Mindful Approach to Managing Your Media Consumption 65

The Benefits and Drawbacks of Instant-access Media 66

Introducing a Mindful Approach to Managing Your Media Consumption 68

Remember: 72

About Annemarie Wiegand 73

PART 2 PRACTISING SELF-CARE, COMPASSION AND KINDNESS 75

9 Mindful Yoga 77

What is Yoga? 78

What is Mindful Yoga? 78
Breathing 79
When is a Good Time to Practise Yoga? 80
Tips for Mindful Yoga Practice 81
How to Practise Mindful Yoga 82
Remember: 85
About Jamila Knopp 86

10 Mindful Eating 87
Considering Your Relationship with Food 88
Mindful Eating 89
Mindful Food Shopping and Preparation 90
Don't Forget to Get a Drink 91
Forbidden Fruit 92
Remember: 93
About Lucie Kysučanová 94

11 Showing Ourselves Compassion 95
Bringing Mindfulness to Self-Compassion During Challenging Times 96
A Self-Compassion Practice 99
Remember: 101
About Stephanie Sackerman 102

12 Growing Gratitude 103
Understanding Dissatisfaction 104
Mindfully Focusing on Gratitude 105
Gratitude Practices 106

Gratitude Tips.. 109

Remember: 110

About Laura Goren.. 111

13 The Power of Being Kind to Others 113

The Gift of Taking Action.. 114

The Role of Perception in Being Kind 116

The Benefits of Being Kind 118

Remember: 120

About Sara Winiecki 121

14 Micro-mindfulness Moments: Mindful Cleaning......... 123

Finding Ways to Look After Yourself 124

Mindful Cleaning 126

Personal Hygiene... 128

Remember: 130

About Cheryl Green 131

15 Mindfulness for Finding Joy 133

Enabling the Conditions Where Joy Exists and Grows....... 134

Remember: 138

About Jennifer Gilroy... 139

16 Connecting with Nature 141

What Is Nature Connection? 141

Where Does Mindfulness Come into It? 142

Why Practise Mindful Nature Connection? 143

Some Suggested Practices.. 144

Finding a Natural Mindfulness Guide 146

Remember: 147
About Clare Snowdon 148

17 Mindful Movement in Nature 149
Brand New Day 149
About Lauretta Mazza 152

PART 3 CONNECTING MINDFULLY WITH OTHERS 153

18 Mindful Communication in Challenging Times 155
Communicating during a Crisis 156
Cultivating Presence 156
The Seeds of Mindful Communication 157
Remember: 162
About Calvin Niles 164

19 Connecting with Others Online 165
Awareness 167
Acceptance 170
Creativity 170
Remember: 172
About Melissa Acuna-Dengo 174

20 Mindful Ways to Work from Home 175
Routine, Routine, Routine! 176
Set Boundaries 178
Moving, Moments and Meditation 179
Reach Out 181
Be Grateful, and Be Kind to Yourself 181
Remember: 183

About Yvonne Cookson 184
21 Staying Mindful with Difficult People 185
   Four Friends 186
   Automatic Thoughts versus Thinking 187
   Being Mindful of Thoughts, Feelings and Actions: Going beyond Positive Thinking.. 189
   Dealing Mindfully with Difficult People 191
   Remember: 193
   About Shabbir Ahmed and Shraddha Shah 194
22 Mindful Ways through Conflict 195
   Be Accepting 196
   Conflict in the Body 197
   Check in with Your Feelings Using HALT 197
   Be Curious about Conflict 198
   Soothe the Conflict Within 199
   Remember: 201
   About Tosh Brittan 202
23 Parenting Mindfully through Challenges 203
   Noticing/Awareness 205
   Allowing... 207
   Acceptance 210
   Remember: 212
   About Crysal Olds 213
24 Mindful Co-parenting and Single Parenting 215
   Recognising the Challenges 216

Responding Mindfully 217
Coping Techniques for Single Parents and Co-parents in Times of Crisis 220
Stories of Hope and Appreciation 222
Remember: 223
About Elspeth Lewis 224

25 Mindfulness for Helping Professionals 225
Responding to Your Own Thoughts and Feelings 225
How Mindfulness Can Help Us Care for Ourselves 228
Remember: 233
About Karen Whitehead 234

26 Mindfulness for Empathy Fatigue 235
What's the Difference between Sympathy, Empathy and Compassion? 236
Understanding Empathy Fatigue and How to Combat It 237
Unlocking the Benefits of Mindfulness 238
Remember: 240
About Michelle Alberigi McKenzie 241

Appendix Audio Tracks 243

Bibliography 247

Dedication

This book is dedicated to all the key workers around the world, risking their lives to save ours. Many, many thanks from the bottom of our hearts.

100% of the profits from this book will go to charities and nonprofits that support the health of the planet.

Acknowledgements

A big thank you to each and every author for their kind contribution to this book. And many thanks to Kerry and Rachael for working hard during evenings and weekends to edit the book and get it into shape for a very tight deadline. Thanks to Emily for the cover designs. Thanks to Oprah for preparing the manuscript so it's accessible as an ebook and paperback. And thank you to Teresa and Diana for their work in supporting me to nurture our Teach Mindfulness Graduates and Community over the many years we've worked together.

Foreword

I've known Shamash for a number of years due to my own interest in the positive benefits of mindfulness. I actually realised later that he was the author of the international bestseller *Mindfulness For Dummies,* a book that I had flipped through several times in various bookshops. Mindfulness for many people appears foreign, mysterious and hard. Yet, in a very simple and straightforward fashion, *Mindfulness For Dummies* explained the why and how of mindfulness and the fact that anyone can do it.

When I realised that Shamash had written the book, my admiration for him grew even greater. You see, Shamash is not motivated by fame or fortune; he genuinely wants to give every person tools to improve their lives and to make living this life easier. This has led him to not only author multiple books, but also develop a number of mindfulness programs and to train mindfulness instructors. He is not only a coach to many, but also an inspiration of what is possible when you truly realise your passion.

Over the years, our paths have crossed many times and we have collaborated on multiple projects. In all instances, it has been a delight. A delight to see him at work and a delight to spend time with this wonderful individual and see him just be. In many ways, this book is a manifestation of him being, and the impact that being has on so many others.

It is, indeed, a challenging time for so many. One that can result in immense fear, anxiety and the potential to spiral into depression. *Mindfulness for Challenging Times: A Collection of Voices for Peace, Self-care and Connection* is a comprehensive volume that gives an overview of mindfulness and highlights its power to address pretty much all those challenges that will arise in times such as these. And one of the great things about this volume is that each chapter is written by a mindfulness teacher who Shamash has trained. Essentially, every chapter has a piece of Shamash in it.

I believe this volume will not only remind those experienced in mindfulness of its many benefits, but also will serve as a roadmap to many who may not yet have any experience or understand the value of mindfulness. And remember, these techniques have been with us for thousands of years. The reason? They work!

I hope you enjoy this volume as much as I have.

James R. Doty, MD

Founder and Director, The Stanford Center for Compassion and Altruism Research and Education (CCARE)

The New York Times bestselling author of *Into the Magic Shop: A Neurosurgeon's Quest to Discover the Mysteries of the Brain and the Secrets of the Heart*

The Story Behind This Book

The idea for this book happened spontaneously in my local park. I was talking on a video call with our community of mindfulness teachers who I've trained over the last seven years. On the call, I asked if we could write a book together to help people at this challenging time. Everyone could contribute a chapter each. The teachers could write about whatever they wished. I got a huge positive response. Nearly 30 people said they were willing to write a chapter and many also offered guided audio meditations to go with it. And all of them suggested different chapters. You're holding the fruits of that initial seed.

The authors have kindly gifted their time to share their insights with you. Some were busy home-schooling. Others are going through their own personal challenges. Many have never been published before. And yet, with kindness and courage, they made time and space to contribute. The editors of this book worked over weekends to ensure we could publish the book in time to launch on 16th May 2020 – the United Nations International Day of Living Together in Peace. A beautiful day to launch this book.

The beauty of having different authors sharing their ideas is that you get to hear different opinions and a range of perspectives. And I think shifting perspectives is really healthy. It's so easy to see things from just one angle.

One of our mindfulness teachers, Puja, sent me this uplifting story of how her work as a mindfulness teacher has both helped her and others:

Sharing mindfulness during this time with the coronavirus has been really fulfilling for me. I was able to restart meditation at our global organisation, which has been specialising in fighting HIV, TB and malaria for years. The online mindfulness classes have allowed many staff to join in. I guide a short meditation on Tuesday and Thursday mornings, and my heart is joyful when I hear back from staff saying how helpful it has been to start the day mindfully, being grounded and focused. Being originally from Nepal, I have also made time to spread mindfulness to fifty women entrepreneurs in Nepal. They were so keen to learn mindfulness and reap the benefits after just three sessions. Thank you so much.

If you would like to find out more about our Teach Mindfulness community, send an email to info@shamashalidina.com, or visit our websites, TeachMindfulnessOnline.com for our teacher training program, or ShamashAlidina.com for our weekly blog.

Introduction

How to Use Mindfulness in Challenging Times

Shamash Alidina

If you've picked up this book, you're probably going through a hard time. Maybe you've lost your job. Perhaps you're struggling in your personal relationships. Loneliness or loss may be a huge challenge for you, or maybe you're feeling deeply overwhelmed by all the changes that surround you.

Whatever the challenge, firstly remember: you're not alone. Whatever challenge you're facing, we're hoping the words in this book will offer you some peace. Although not everyone is suffering, these certainly are challenging times for millions of people. You're not alone in your suffering. Reflecting that we are all in this together can help.

Secondly, appreciate the difference between pain and suffering. Your challenges may be causing you pain right now. And we all experience pain at some time. It can be the physical pain of an injury or illness, or the emotional pain of a loss or change. But in mindfulness, we distinguish between pain and suffering.

Pain is inevitable. But suffering is different. Suffering is what arises when you struggle to accept what can't be changed; when, instead of accepting, you deny, fight or even reject your present moment experience.

Acceptance is not easy. That's why so many of us are not only experiencing pain, but also suffering.

Acceptance comes in its own time. But sometimes, mindful approaches can help you along that journey. The authors in this book offer you different ways to be mindful and accept what's happening in your life. Not an acceptance that's giving up or tolerating. But an acceptance that's empowering, life-affirming and calming. An acceptance that makes you feel like you're rising to the challenge. An acceptance that is born out of self-care and kindness.

There are many misconceptions about mindfulness. They can lead to unnecessary struggles, and so I'd like to clarify the concept. Mindfulness is not about trying to relax. It's not about thinking positively. And it's not about making your mind blank. Then what is it? It's about simply being present with what is. Being open to your moment-to-moment experience with acceptance, kindness and curiosity. No silent mind is required. So you can do it, and you can bring your crazy mind along with you – it's very welcome. You can be mindful in this way right now, and you can also do the mindful meditations to deepen your experience.

Whatever happens, please don't feel that you're doing anything wrong in your response to your challenges. It's really hard when the whole of society is turned upside down. Everyone's response is slightly different, and your response isn't bad or wrong. Maybe you don't feel like doing anything. Or perhaps you're going into work overdrive. Maybe you feel overwhelmed by the sorrow the world faces.

Begin by acknowledging that these are really hard times; the toughest that society has faced in half a century. So, of course, your body and mind are going to struggle and respond in ways that seem wrong. That's ok. Being kind to yourself and accepting yourself as you are is very much part of the spirit of being mindful. Imperfection isn't our enemy – it's what makes us human.

Mindfulness doesn't offer any quick fixes. But a moment of presence can help you to see your challenge in a totally different way – and that can sometimes change everything. The potential for radical transformation in a moment is very much possible.

But mostly, mindfulness offers you another option. Another way to relate to the difficulties you're encountering. Right now, perhaps when you feel overwhelmed or stressed, you may overeat, shout at someone in frustration, or reach for a drink. We're all susceptible to making choices that don't help in the long run. But you may not have the skills or capacity to do anything differently. However, some short mindfulness exercises in this book may be an alternative you choose, both practised in moments of calm or when facing really tough moments.

Tiny changes matter. It's our hope that this book inspires you to take just one deep, mindful breath, in and out. Or one long, much-needed stretch of your body. Or to be a little bit nicer to yourself. There's no pressure to do any more than that. If you're inspired to try more, well, in this challenging time, we'll be very impressed.

If you want to try a mindful reflection now, begin with this exercise. It's a way to step back from your difficulties and potentially receive some guidance that is both wise and kind. You can hear the audio for this exercise at TeachMindfulnessOnline.com/book.

Inner Advisor Reflection

1. Begin by sitting comfortably.
2. Take a few deep, conscious breaths and enjoy the feeling as you breathe in and out, as best as you can.
3. Think of someone who represents wisdom and kindness. It can be someone who's alive or not. It can be a spiritual teacher, or a friend or a family member you respect.
4. Imagine you're with them right now. They smile and you smile back, feeling at ease in their presence.
5. Tell them about your challenge. Watch them listening to you. And listen to any advice they have for you.
6. Continue your conversation for as long as you wish, in your imagination.
7. Thank them when you've finished and reflect on what you heard.
8. Bring this exercise slowly to an end, and spend a couple of minutes writing down your reflections.

Was the advice you received helpful? If so, are you able to put any of that advice into practice, now or in the future?

How to Use This Book

In these challenging times, we want this book and audio to be a support rather than an extra burden for you. Whether you've tried mindfulness before, or you're considering trying it for the first time, begin with short, simple exercises. Dip in and out, or read as many chapters of this book that you feel able to.

Here's one approach. Start with some everyday mindfulness – being conscious of your day-to-day activities. Then try the short guided mindfulness meditations. Go for the longer meditations when you're ready to dive in – but there's no rush.

Remember, this book is not a replacement for medical advice. If you're feeling overwhelmed, please seek out professional advice. If you don't know who to talk to, visit www.befrienders.org, or call the Befrienders or Samaritans in your country. They can provide confidential, emotional support, no matter what the cause of suffering.

Listening to guided mindfulness audio tracks is a great way to practise mindfulness for most people. To freely access all the guided mindfulness audio tracks that go with this book (plus bonus tracks), go to TeachMindfulnessOnline.com/book. You can find a full list of the audio tracks in the Appendix.

About Shamash Alidina

Shamash is the author of *Mindfulness For Dummies* and *The Mindful Way Through Stress*, and the co-founder of the Museum of Happiness in London. He offers Mindfulness Teacher Training and Acceptance and Commitment Training, both fully online. He's currently very passionate about the philosophy of non-duality. He's based in London, UK.

ShamashAlidina.com

PART 1
MEETING CHALLENGES WITH MINDFULNESS

1

Finding Calm in the Chaos

Dawn Andrews

When a crisis strikes, how can we prepare ourselves? How can we cope when we are in the thick of it? What tools can we use to ensure we come through relatively intact, and how do we pick ourselves up quickly afterwards?

You'll find some possible answers to these questions in this chapter, as well as a simple and effective mindfulness practice that you can do at any time.

This chapter has been written in the middle of the coronavirus pandemic. A time of crisis, if ever there was one. It all happened so fast that no one escaped the shell-shock. One-minute things were ticking along okay, and then, suddenly, everything changed.

Now, we are all stuck at home in lockdown: maybe home-schooling the kids, or wondering how to fill the time off work, or perhaps awaiting the next payslip to see if the reduced wages will cover the bills.

Then there's the person who's lost their job. The small business that's lost most of their customers. And the self-employed person having to seek benefits for the first time in their life.

People now working from home are getting under their partner's feet, family members are disturbing home workers when they're in full flow, and then there's the unfamiliarity of working alone without a team. It all feels strange, uncomfortable, difficult. So much tension, concern, worry, fear, anxiety, stress, uncertainty.

As if that wasn't enough, we are also cut off from our support network of our family and friends, missing out on all that good-feeling oxytocin. While all those 'what-ifs' are screaming at us, we can't even get a hug from our parents or siblings!

The physical outcomes of a crisis can become obvious; for instance, lack of sleep, anxiety, panic attacks or agoraphobia. If we are sufficiently aware of these, we can start to address them before they become major issues.

But what about the mental health outcomes? In a time of crisis, our stress levels are likely to go through the roof, our thoughts can be confusing and erratic, and our emotions can range from feeling afraid to feeling angry or frustrated, guilty, lonely, helpless, anxious, devastated, sad or worried.

Any go-to coping mechanisms we have will have been tested to the hilt. How do we stop our thoughts and feelings from overwhelming us – at least long enough to enable us to adapt to the situation?

This is where mindfulness can help save the day in any crisis.

How Mindfulness Can Help

The Oxford Dictionary states mindfulness is "a mental state achieved by focusing one's awareness on the present moment, while calmly acknowledging and accepting one's feelings, thoughts, and bodily sensations".

If you are left wondering how that could help us in a crisis, consider these two important points.

Firstly, it has been shown that for nearly half of our day we are not really present. It's true. Two students from Harvard created an app called 'Track Your Happiness', which tracked people's everyday activities to gauge their level of happiness. The research proved that, on average, our minds wander about 47 per cent of the time. And, for most of that time, we are not happy, as we are either worrying about the past or concerned about the future.

Secondly, bear in mind the Buddhist parable of the 'second arrow', which states there are two kinds of suffering: the actual pain of a situation, and the worry and stress we layer over the top of it.

So, if we can put more of that 47 per cent to better use, and recognise and soothe that second layer, we would be so much better equipped to cope in a crisis! And mindfulness can help us to do just that.

When we focus our awareness on the present moment, rather than the past or future, we arrive at a calm, still space within where our mind isn't wandering so much. We can therefore start to reclaim some of that 47 per cent.

Then, while in this calm space, we can gently get in touch with and observe those worrisome thoughts, feelings and bodily sensations. We can allow them to exist, and begin to accept them with kindness and compassion, instead of pushing them aside. This helps to soothe that second layer.

The more we practise mindfulness, the better equipped we become to make wiser, less emotive decisions, enabling us to *choose* how we respond.

A Little Neuroscience

Within the brain is:

- **The cortex** (top part of the head): The thought processor.
- **The prefrontal cortex** (the forehead): Where good judgements are made.
- **The amygdala** (in the middle of the head): Where raw emotions are stored.

When a crisis comes along, we judge the situation, which determines the level of stress and fear we attach to it.

Within this process, the cortex looks for similar memories, and the amygdala offers up the emotions that match it. Then, the prefrontal cortex helps make judgements from those memories and emotions.

If the prefrontal cortex is strong, it helps us make good judgements in clarity. This reduces the possibility of stress.

If the prefrontal cortex is not so strong, judgements are less clear. Stress levels then begin to rise, and if they keep rising, the body can go into overdrive. This is how you end up with fight/flight/freeze – anxiety and panic. And in this state, it is hard to cope in a crisis.

The good news is that practising mindfulness strengthens the prefrontal cortex.

Changing Our Perception

The way we think about stress matters too. We can perceive stress differently by recognising it as our friend, rather than an enemy. Which really, if we think about it, is actually true.

The body doesn't produce symptoms related to stress because it doesn't like us. It produces these symptoms to take care of us. It says, "Hey, please notice that you are potentially overloading the system. Please review your thought processes to reduce your level of stress!"

It's giving us a sign, asking us to adapt to meet the challenge differently. And when we do, we soon realise that we really can trust ourselves to handle life's challenges. We recognise – we've got this!

PACE: A Mindfulness Practice

Here's a simple mindfulness exercise for you to practise to find calm amid the chaos (you can involve your whole family if you wish). It only takes three or four minutes. In this practice you will PACE: **P**osition, become **A**ware, **C**heck in and **E**mbrace.

Mindfulness is all about being gentle with ourselves. You are just giving yourself a minute, for you, amidst all the chaos. There is no need to adopt a perfect cross-legged posture (unless you wish to, that is). You can sit, stand or lie down for this exercise.

So, let's start by taking a few long... slow... deep breaths. Really take your time with each breath. Just a few deep breaths, to help you to relax. And after a few breaths, just bring your breath back to its natural rhythm.

Then, when you are ready, *position* one hand on your stomach, and the other hand on your chest. As you do this, start to notice which hand is rising as you breathe. Is it the one on your chest, or the one on your stomach? Give yourself a moment to notice.

If it is the chest, next time you breathe in, try to draw the breath through your stomach instead. Notice your stomach rising underneath your hand. It can take a bit of getting used to, so allow yourself a minute or so to notice. Just breathing through the stomach, not the chest.

Don't worry if you suddenly start breathing through the chest again. You may have been breathing this way for some time. It takes practice. Just, when you notice, draw your breath through your stomach again. And continue doing this for a little while. You will soon notice you feel calmer.

Keeping your hands in place, gently become *aware* of your thoughts, feelings and bodily sensations. Just allow yourself to notice whatever you are thinking, how you are feeling, and which bodily sensations you may be experiencing.

You don't want to get embroiled in the story of your thoughts. You just want to become aware of the thoughts being there, and then give them a moment to have their say, while noticing if there are any feelings and bodily sensations attached to these thoughts.

Maybe you feel some tension in your shoulders, or your forehead may be creased. Perhaps your jaw feels tight. Or maybe there's some tightness in your stomach.

If you don't notice any feelings or sensations, that's okay too. It's perfectly normal if you don't.

So, you are just giving yourself a little time to notice. A minute or so is fine, just to have an idea of what is going on for you, right now, in this moment.

When you are ready, let go of your attention on the thoughts, feelings and sensations, and *check in* with where your hands are. If the hand on your chest is rising, just bring your attention to the hand on your stomach. Again, drawing your breath through your stomach and noticing your hand rising. Keep with this for a minute or so. Now you are getting the hang of it. Can you notice that you are feeling more calm and clear?

So, let's take it one step further.

In this calm place, ask yourself, what one thing can you do differently to *embrace* this challenge that you are in?

Just a simple, manageable, baby step that you know you can do to help ease this situation, and reduce your worry load.

Take a moment to reflect, until you find that one baby step you know you can do, right now.

Now – go and do it.

Remember:

- We will always experience crises in our lives, but we can respond mindfully to them.
- Practising mindfulness can strengthen the prefrontal cortex and help us find clarity.
- Use the mindfulness exercise **P**osition, **A**ware, **C**heck in and **E**mbrace to find a moment of calm amidst the chaos.

About Dawn Andrews

Dawn is a mindfulness teacher and CBT coach. She is based in Devon, UK.

www.mindfullyu.co.uk

2

Staying Mindful in Isolation

Terry McCoy

We all need to feel a sense of connection and belonging. Research has shown that even a *perceived* lack of belonging can make us feel anxious. Being in isolation during the coronavirus pandemic may have been testing your feelings of belonging.

In this chapter, I share a few practical mindfulness tips to help if you are feeling anxious from the emotional strain of isolation.

Connect

When home isolation was introduced in the UK during the pandemic, mutual aid groups appeared on social media within 24 hours offering to pick up shopping for vulnerable people or provide their time to phone someone on their own; an outstanding example of the need to band together, communicate and connect to help others. When this situation is resolved, I hope that this sense of community will continue and grow. Whether or not it does is up to us. If you're self-isolating on your own, make the decision now to *connect*. Talk with a friend, a family member (pretend you like them), or a work colleague. Get in touch by phone or using a video app. Make it part of your day. Decide to connect with two other people every day.

Be Selective, Be a Detective

"We are more often frightened than hurt, and we suffer more in imagination than in reality." Seneca

Social media is a handy way to stay connected. However, there's a lot of scaremongering and misinformation on there. It seems to be worse since the coronavirus raised its spiky little head, adding to the feelings of anxiety, fear and uncertainty.

Be mindful of what you choose to read. If you read something upsetting and you have a tendency to worry, check the facts. For example, according to a recent video, breathing in hot air from a hairdryer will kill the coronavirus (I kid you not). Exercise digital media literacy: a quick search on independent fact-checking websites (such as Snopes.com or FactCheck.org) shows that the information is false. It was just hot air (no pun intended) – but how many people have the added anxiety caused by burnt lips?

A way to alleviate fear and uncertainty is to get the facts. Learn to discern.

When you read something that doesn't feel right or provokes a strong adverse reaction:

1. Put down or move away from your device.
2. Ask yourself, "What do I feel right now?"
3. Label the feeling. When we can put a label to an emotion or feeling, it can help to disable it. If you are unsure of the feeling, then give it a colour: what's important is that you know what the colour means.

This technique creates a 'change space' between you and the emotion, so rather than react impulsively, you can choose to respond. You are at a choice point here, so take responsibility before you believe or share the content.

Pay Attention to What You Can Control

"We should always be asking ourselves: 'Is this something that is, or is not, in my control?'" *Epictetus*

This quote is taken from stoic philosophy, which you can find out more about online. One of the most useful components of this philosophy is about control, and differentiating between what we can and can't control.

There are many factors that are uncertain and that are simply beyond our control. This can change in a heartbeat. Our lives can change in a moment. And that's always been the case and always will be. Uncertainty is the only thing we can be sure of at present.

"Trust God and tie up your camels" is an old saying, which means do what you can in each situation and let go of the rest. One antidote to feeling a lack of control or certainty is to focus on what you can control. You may have heard this before – the following exercise shows you how you can put that into practice.

Ask yourself:

- "What can I control/do in this situation?"
- "What are my choices here?"

Try this 21-day experiment to give you a plan of action. Starting tonight, before you go to sleep, write down three things you can do in the next 24 hours. For some, it might be spending an hour learning the ukulele that's been sitting in your wardrobe for two years. For others, it might be going for a walk around the block.

Doing this activity gives you something to focus on, increases your sense of control and degree of certainty, and decreases your level of anxiety.

The three things you pick are not written in stone. You can change your mind the next morning if you want to; it's your choice.

Mindfulness in Motion

Try these fun mindfulness exercises while you are at home.

Mindfulness in motion for the children (and you can join in):

1. Fill a paper cup three-quarters full of cold water and have the children pass the cup clockwise to the next person. Let them get accustomed to the game. They will be bored within minutes.
2. Ask them to do the same thing, but this time with their eyes closed and no talking.
3. Reverse direction. You may think this is a recipe for chaos, but you would be surprised. In eight years, I can only

remember two or three spillages – and all but one were from adults!

Create your own mindfulness in motion activity:

1. *Involve as many of the five senses as possible, or at least sight, sound and touch.*
2. *Make it rhythmic and fun.*
3. *Make it scalable. Too easy, and it becomes boring. Too challenging, and it becomes stressful.*

I share a guided audio meditation that may serve as an antidote to isolation, which you may like to try: visit TeachMindfulnessOnline.com/book.

Remember:

- Connect with others every day to enhance your feelings of community and belonging.
- Be mindful when reading news stories.
- Pay attention to what you can control during isolation.

About Terry McCoy

Terry teaches practical mindfulness, which includes formal and informal mindfulness activities, as well as drawing from other disciplines and the belief systems of stoic philosophy and Buddhism. He is based in Liverpool, England.

www.thenlpworks.com

3

Finding Ways to Cope with Stress

Pierpaolo Paparo

We all experience stress. It's part of what makes us human. But what causes stress? *Stress* is any change that occurs to your mind or body as a result of coping with a change to your life.

Stress is not necessarily a bad thing; on the contrary, a moderate amount of stress makes life more enjoyable. Whether you're engaged in a competition, confronting a difficult situation at work or experiencing a major life-changing event, you will experience a stress response, and you will then try to adapt to this response.

Managing stress is not about reducing stress; instead, it is about being able to return to a state of ease after a stressful event has occurred. Similarly, managing stress effectively can help you cope even in the middle of a major life-changing event. 'Bad' or 'chronic' stress arises when you lose this ability to reduce your level of stress, which leads to significant physical and emotional distress.

Your Body's Response to Stress

You may have noticed that when you face a challenge, your body reacts. When you encounter what your mind interprets to be 'danger' (whether this is real or imagined), you activate your stress response and you move into a state of fight/flight. Your body gets ready to respond to the danger: your heart rate increases, your breathing speeds up and your blood pressure may rise. Once the danger has passed, your body is able to turn on its relaxation response, and you ease into the rest/digest state. In this state, your breathing is easy, your heart rate and blood pressure go back to normal, and you experience calm.

Transitions from the fight/flight response and back to the rest/digest state are normal and healthy. However, chronic stress arises when the stress response stays in place for a prolonged period due to challenging life circumstances. Chronic stress can also build up over time if you experience a number of stress-inducing events that you struggle to fully recover from.

What Are the Key Sources of Stress?

The coronavirus pandemic is an example of an environmental stressor. During a crisis such as a pandemic, everybody – from individuals through to small and large organisations, entire governments and countries – has to adapt to a new way of living. So your *environment* can be a source of stress. Other examples of environmental stressors include an unexpected noise from outside when you are asleep, pollution or even earthquakes or floods.

Other people can be the cause of your stress too! These are called *social* stressors. An argument with your boss, financial issues, domestic chores or a change in the family household structure can all cause you to feel stressed.

Even your own thought process (a *psychological* stressor) can be a significant source of stress. Often your beliefs about your ability to cope with a given situation can create more stress than the situation itself!

Through mindfulness, you can see how your belief in the stories you tell yourself in your mind, can cause you stress. Thoughts like 'I'm not good enough', or 'I hate this situation – I can't stand it'. These unhelpful thoughts about ourselves, others and the world can trigger the stress response.

From clearly seeing that these responses are just thoughts and not necessarily facts, may arise a call for you to act: to make the changes you want to make, but also to accept the things that you cannot change. You will be able to act from a place of clarity.

Near the beginning of my career, when working for a financial institution, I experienced high levels of anxiety. Only after starting on a path of meditation and self-discovery, could I clearly see that most of the anxiety was coming from my belief in my own thoughts. I assumed all my thoughts to be true – but they were just passing ideas that I was taking too seriously! It took me a while to see my thoughts as just thoughts, and when I did so, my level of anxiety dropped considerably.

Notice what thoughts you're having that may be causing you stress, and try to see them as just that – thoughts that you can allow to come and go like clouds in the sky, without having to take them so seriously.

Healthy and Unhealthy Ways to Cope with Stress

There are several ways you can try to cope with stress. Some of the most common 'unhealthy' ways include eating more than usual (or more than needed), working longer hours, withdrawing emotionally, increasing alcohol or tobacco consumption, sleeping in or going to bed late, buying things just to get a momentary thrill, and taking sleeping pills.

Fortunately, you can also take a healthier approach to managing stress. Healthier strategies include improving your social interactions, doing more physical exercise, getting involved in new hobbies, and maintaining a healthy diet. If the situation that is causing you stress is external (such as an environmental or social stressor) you can go ahead and try to change it; and if the situation is one you cannot change, you can practise accepting the situation using mindfulness.

Another effective strategy to help you deal with stressful situations is to practise some simple mindful exercises that allow you to increase your awareness of your thought processes and help you see your challenging experience in a different light.

Mindful Exercises to Help Ease Stress

These exercises are quick tension-releasers and are a great place to start if you want to manage your stress levels and take better care of yourself.

Any type of stress response exercise should be practised regularly, ideally daily, to provide a long-term beneficial effect. You are slowly rewiring your entire nervous system for better mental health, and repetition is of fundamental importance for this rewiring to be a success.

Remember, do these exercises with the spirit of mindfulness. That means being aware of the sensations, being accepting of whatever happens, and being kind to your body and mind. The aim is not that you *must* relieve your stress or tension – that can cause more stress! Instead, the aim is just to experiment and see what happens when you try these approaches.

Grounding (5–10 seconds)

This grounding exercise can last from five to ten seconds, and you can do it whenever you feel your stress response starting to kick in. You can perform it while you're sitting at your desk, standing still or even talking to somebody.

1. You may be sitting or standing, but not lying down. Your feet should be in contact with the ground.
2. As soon you notice a feeling of tension arise, or you start ruminating about an issue that has been on your mind, bring your attention to your feet. Make sure they are on the ground.
3. Rest your attention on the sensation of your feet touching the ground, whether directly or through the soles of your shoes. If it helps, move your feet slightly and notice any change in sensation or change in your balance. Five to ten seconds is enough.

4. When you've finished, return to what you were doing before you started the exercise.

Shaking your body (10–20 seconds)

In this exercise, you are going to shake the tension from your body. You can practise this exercise at any time during the day when your body feels tense. You must be standing.

1. While standing, shake your arms and legs as athletes do before an important competition. Shake your body for 10–20 seconds.
2. After the exercise, notice any change in tension in your body. Be curious.

Stamping your feet (10 seconds)

You can practise this exercise at any time, while sitting or standing. It is a remarkably effective tension releaser for some. (This makes some noise, so you might not be able to do it everywhere!)

1. As you are sitting or standing, stamp your feet quickly on the floor. Do this for around ten seconds.
2. After the exercise, notice any changes in your body or mind.

With all of these short exercises, bring as much curiosity as you can to the experience. Be open, engaged and playful if you can. Relaxation is a welcome side-effect rather than the goal.

Remember:

- Stress is a normal and healthy response. However, prolonged periods of chronic stress are harmful to your mind and body.
- Healthy strategies for managing stress include eating well, exercising, taking part in new hobbies and activities, and socialising. If personal contact with others is a challenge (for example, due to physical distancing), try using video and audio calls to stay in touch with people.
- Engaging in even short mindful exercises can help you meet your challenges with curiosity, openness and acceptance.

About Pierpaolo Paparo

Pierpaolo is a certified mindfulness teacher and a graduate of psychotherapy and counselling. His aim is to facilitate self-discovery and wholeness by integrating learnings coming from meditation, spirituality and psychology. He's based in Dublin, Ireland.

www.selfdiscoveryways.com

4

Mindfulness for Anxiety

Caitriona Horan

I want to share with you the benefits of mindfulness in lowering the effects of anxiety. I first took up formal mindfulness as an antidote to workplace stress, and, as my practice deepened, I became aware of anxiety that had been with me most of my life. I realised that I had been creating mindful coping methods for myself long before I had ever heard the word 'mindfulness'.

My formal mindfulness journey took me from lecturing in management studies to becoming a mindfulness teacher and life coach. I have witnessed how mindfulness builds up resilience in my clients and in myself. *Resilience* is our ability to deal with, find strength in and recover from difficulty; our ability to 'bounce back' more quickly, which is invaluable during the crisis situations we all experience both individually and collectively.

The resilience promoted by mindfulness practice and meditation means fewer 'wobbles' and faster recovery from them as we build a stronger connection with the calm place we all have within us. My hope is that something in this chapter may resonate with you, helping you to connect more closely with your own inner calm.

Remember, follow the advice and guidance of your doctors, especially if you have a medically diagnosed anxiety disorder.

What is Anxiety?

Anxiety is a natural feeling of fear, worry or tension that we all have from time to time, often when we feel threatened by a stressful event. Small, sometimes unnoticed stressful situations can build up and distress us mentally or physically, as most of us will have experienced to some extent. However, when the fight/flight/freeze response (a protection mechanism explained in detail in Chapter 6) is switched on most of the time it can affect everyday functioning, cause unhappiness and impair mental health. At times of crisis, rapid change can make us feel anxious.

Anxiety is also connected to overthinking 'what-ifs', and there is a clear distinction between planning for different future scenarios in a practical way and worrying about all the things that might go wrong. Unfortunately, our minds have evolved a protective 'negativity-bias' that causes us to think in this way. You may have heard the quote attributed to Mark Twain: "I am an old man and have known a great many troubles, but most of them never happened." We experience anxiety through our thoughts, emotions and physical sensations around something in the near or distant future that we believe will, or could, happen. The subconscious mind and the body respond in the same way whether the fear is of something real (that is happening now) or imaginary (in the future). Telling ourselves that our fears are irrational simply does not work – ask anyone who has a phobia of, say, mice or spiders!

Being impatient with ourselves and telling ourselves to 'get a grip', or worse, is not at all helpful. Sometimes we fight and suppress seemingly 'undesirable' emotions like anxiety, but this suppression merely hides them. They may emerge unexpectedly later as they are ancient reactions programmed into our brains over millennia when survival depended on outwitting predators.

Perhaps the most disturbing manifestation of anxiety is experiencing a panic attack. This can be confusing, as the 'fight/flight/freeze' response may be triggered unexpectedly, resulting in fear and distressing physical symptoms such as a pounding heart. It is not always clear to us what the fear is about – and it could simply be fear of the unknown itself, especially in times of crisis. At night-time, particularly, panic can seem more intense and less manageable. Perhaps our feelings are amplified in the darkness without the distraction of our other senses, such as sight and sound.

Remember that challenging times are always temporary. We have all experienced times when our world seemed to have been turned upside down. We have lost people through death, divorce or distancing. We have lost money and possessions. We have changed jobs or schools or accommodation. Whatever the change, we have somehow coped with it, as we all have the inner resources to deal with changes great or small.

Reading words on a page and knowing that anxiety is a common and shared human state, for which we all have the coping resources, may not magically help us with our own anxiety. But mindfulness can make a real and lasting difference.

How Does Mindfulness Help with Anxiety?

Rather than fighting difficult emotions such as anxiety, which have a positive protective purpose, mindfulness helps us to accept them and respond in a more positive way with self-compassion. Through mindfulness, we gradually realise and accept that thoughts, emotions and physical feelings are passing events that may be here one moment and gone the next: "This too shall pass." The concept of acceptance is very important to mindfulness. It doesn't mean that we have to submit to a situation we feel is wrong for us, such as being lonely, trapped or experiencing loss. It simply means we accept that this is what we are experiencing now. There will be better moments. The uncomfortable thoughts, emotions and physical sensations have simply come to visit us for a while. The idea of being visited by and even welcoming difficult emotions, such as anxiety, is beautifully addressed in the poem *The Guest House* by the 13th-century mystic, Rumi, which you can search for online.

If it seems alien to welcome an unwanted guest like anxiety, you could consider simply thanking your mind for trying to protect you. Anxiety is a visitor that has come for a reason, and you could ask the emotion what it is bringing to you.

During a recent tragic family crisis, I practised saying, "Hello anxiety, my old friend." Although it was a heartbreaking, frightening and difficult time, being able to detach from the anxiety and view it as a visitor somehow helped me to perform the practical and supportive tasks that were needed. Detachment is about knowing that you and the anxiety are not the same. You are not the anxiety; you're merely experiencing anxiety. The core holistic 'YOU' is a lot more than this anxiety, which is evident in the fact that you can observe it.

The Science Behind Dealing with Anxiety

The founder of compassion-focussed therapy, world-renowned psychologist Professor Paul Gilbert, describes three emotional regulation systems: the *drive* system that helps you to accomplish tasks and achieve goals; the *soothing* system that helps you to slow down and rest; and the *threat* system that helps you to protect yourself against danger.

The need to balance these three systems is very important for wellbeing. Anxiety belongs to the threat and self-protective system, which triggers the fight/flight/freeze response of stress. Our brains have evolved for survival as opposed to happiness, where protective emotions and thoughts easily override positive ones. The body responds more quickly to threat than to pleasure; we focus on the threat and drive systems most of the time, while neglecting the soothing system.

It is natural to turn towards the drive system when feeling anxious, and taking some sort of action can be good at balancing threat. Exercising can help to reduce anxiety, as can tackling procrastination (such as paying bills or processing paperwork). Action can also take the form of practical mindfulness, such as mindful tea-making, eating (Chapter 10) or hand-washing (Chapter 14) – any activity that absorbs us in the present for however short a time. Taking action can give us a sense of achievement and make us feel good, but it can also become addictive.

We need to consciously promote the positive emotions associated with the soothing system (contentment, feeling safe) in order to maintain balance. Mindful meditation, be it sitting, lying, walking or through some other movement, can feed the soothing system, as can practising self-compassion. It is okay to feel lost, vulnerable, frightened or upset, especially at times of crisis. Mindfulness is not about eliminating normal feelings but recognising them and empathising with ourselves.

Techniques for Soothing Anxious Thoughts

If you are new to the meditation aspect of mindfulness, a gentle approach is recommended in a crisis situation, so start with short guided meditations that focus on the body and simple breathing exercises to help you cope with any anxiety. Regular practice, even a few minutes a day, will gradually build up resilience over time.

Many people find a daily 'body scan' meditation helpful, and I can also personally vouch for its effectiveness following a night-time panic attack. The body scan involves paying attention to each part of your body from your toes up to your head, and observing how it is, as if you are moving a spotlight to each part in turn. I share a guided body scan meditation for you to try: visit TeachMindfulnessOnline.com/book.

With experience, you will be able to carry it out in your mind without any guided audio track and make it your own, as long or short as you wish. I carry out quick 'body scans' throughout the day as I work, just to check in on how my body is feeling and adjust my posture or take a break. Soothing the body also helps soothe the mind. The body scan serves to bring your mind into the present moment and calm down any sense of something being wrong. Your body is always in the present moment, although your mind may wander elsewhere.

Observing your breathing and practising a few slow deep breaths can help with the physical effects of anxiety. Developing the habit of deeper, slower breathing over time brings more oxygen to our brains, promoting clearer, calmer thought. Do not, however, force this. In mindfulness we are never trying to achieve anything, we're simply observing what is. By observing the breath, it may naturally adjust. Remember that our bodies know how to breathe all by themselves.

There are, however, some soothing techniques that you can use when feeling anxious. In crisis situations, an exercise called *square breathing* is often used by military or emergency services personnel. You breathe in for a count of four, hold your breath for a count of four, breathe out for a count of four and wait for a count of four before breathing in again. Another technique is called *4–7–8*, also known as *relaxing breath*, and involves breathing in for four seconds, holding the breath for seven seconds and exhaling slowly for eight seconds. In fact, breathing out more slowly than the in-breath at any time stimulates a large nerve in the body, the vagus nerve that joins the brain to the heart and abdomen, promoting a calming effect.

Breathing out slowly is like sighing. Any of these techniques practised for as long as is comfortable for you can help engage the soothing system (explained in the previous section). Just one mindful breath is a mini-meditation in itself. I also share a short *mindful pause* guided audio track you might like to try, which combines awareness of body and breath: visit TeachMindfulnessOnline.com/book.

Have fun experimenting as you develop your mindfulness practice. The beauty of mindfulness is that any of the exercises or techniques in this book or any you create yourself will contribute to your emotional balance and wellbeing. Be comfortable, be curious, have fun experimenting, be kind to yourself and be happy.

Remember:

- Anxiety is a normal part of being human. It is an emotion that is there to protect us from danger, but if we experience it habitually it can affect our health. Rather than fighting it, accept it as a temporary event. **Throughout your life, you've already courageously navigated many challenges.**

- Mindfulness helps us to build up resilience that enables us to avert or recover quickly from future anxious episodes. Kindness and self-compassion play a big part in this resilience.

- Practising regular mindful action or soothing meditation improves our wellbeing and reduces anxiety. This can simply be for a few minutes several times throughout the day.

About Caitriona Horan

Caitriona Horan, MA, is a certified advanced mindfulness teacher and IAPC&M accredited life coach also offering listening and hypnosis therapies. She's based in Loughton, Essex, UK.

www.behappiest.co.uk

5

Managing Sleep in Challenging Times

Jane Bozier

The alarm goes off and you reach over and hit the snooze button. You think to yourself, "Is it that time already?" You still feel tired and may even feel like you haven't slept. However, whether you're a key worker, home-schooling your children, working from home or self-isolating, you still have to start your day.

You may find that you're struggling to get enough sleep. Here, I share with you some of my own experiences of disrupted sleep, including how the life-changing practices of mindfulness have helped me. I will also talk a little about the science of sleep, bust the myths surrounding sleep, and provide you with some tips to help you experience a more restful night's sleep.

Understanding Your Sleep Cycle

Your sleep cycle (or your *circadian rhythm*) is a 24-hour sleep–wake cycle. Our body clocks are in tune with the light (day) and the dark (night) of each 24-hour cycle thanks to a hormone called melatonin, which the brain releases to regulate our sleep cycle.

When the regular rhythm of each day is disrupted, it can lead to sleep difficulties. To get a sense of why this might be a problem, think back to a time when people lived off the land – a time before electricity and modern-day technology. People went to sleep when it was dark and woke up when it was light. Their body clocks worked with nature. Some people preferred the mornings (the 'larks'), while others preferred the night (the 'owls'). Communities would function well because the larks might choose morning tasks, such as gathering firewood and making breakfast, while the owls might choose evening tasks, such as taking the night watch.

Melatonin is sometimes called the 'sleep hormone'. In today's modern society, many things can interfere with the release of melatonin and therefore affect the quality of our sleep. Artificial light, including the blue light from TVs, smartphones and tablets, can fool the brain into thinking that it is still daytime, which stops the mind and body from preparing for sleep. Your mind may be tired, yet your body is wide awake (or vice versa).

When your circadian rhythm becomes disrupted (such as with jet lag, shift work or a change in your routine), you may struggle to fall asleep, wake frequently, wake early or experience insomnia.

The Stages of Sleep

High-quality sleep is beneficial to overall health and wellbeing. The recommended amount of sleep for an adult is 7–9 hours (babies, children and teenagers require more sleep than adults). A good night's sleep aids memory and concentration, whereas poor sleep is linked to irritability, fatigue and physical diseases such as diabetes and obesity.

Sleep occurs in stages. Stages 1, 2 and 3 are non-rapid eye movement (NREM) sleep stages. Stage 1 is where we transition from being awake to asleep; stage 2 is the intermediate stage before deep sleep occurs, where the heart rate and temperature drop; and stage 3 is where the muscles relax and the blood pressure drops. Stage 4, rapid eye movement (REM) sleep, is where we dream. A complete sleep cycle takes from 90–110 minutes, and we move through these stages of sleep throughout the night.

My Sleep Story

I have always been interested in sleep: what constitutes a good night's sleep, what gets in the way of a good night's sleep and what we can do about it. Understanding that 'one shoe does not fit all' when it comes to sleep patterns and sleep cycles has changed my sleep for the better.

I wake frequently through the night, and I used to feel that I was doing something wrong – I would ask myself constantly why I couldn't do something as natural as fall asleep easily. Unsurprisingly, anxiety would then stop me from going back to sleep. This unhelpful attitude changed through my love of sport and my growing interest in sleep. I came across a book called

Sleep by Nick Littlehales, a leading sleep coach and sleep guru. The book introduced me to R90, or 'recovery in 90 minutes', which is the time it takes to go through a full sleep cycle. Littlehales suggests that keeping a record of the number of cycles that you go through during each night's sleep can help you to set realistic sleep targets. (You can write it down, or use an app such as Peak Sleep – Sleep Better.) Littlehales suggests that instead of aiming for eight hours of uninterrupted sleep, you may be better off aiming for five 90-minute cycles.

I tried this, and my waking through the night no longer became a worry. I was able to fall back to sleep more easily, and when I couldn't achieve the full five cycles, I would be aware of the deficit. At those times, I would try to schedule a power nap into my day until I could get back into my sleep routine.

If you're finding that your sleep is becoming disrupted during difficult times, you may find it helpful to set smaller, more achievable goals to help you manage your sleep such as achieving at least some 90-minute sleep cycles.

Debunking Some Common Myths About Sleep

Here's the real story behind five common beliefs about sleep.

Sleep myth 1: You can get by on little sleep

You can do this occasionally if you need to, but if you cheat on the amount of sleep that you get on a regular basis, it will have a negative impact on your physical and mental health. Poor sleep reduces concentration and overall performance, be it at work or at home. Irritability, anxiety and depression can increase, as can overeating. So, in real terms, it is advisable to put a good night's sleep high on your agenda to remain healthy and happy.

Sleep myth 2: If you wake up in the night, it's best to stay in bed and count sheep

There are two things to talk about here. The first is staying in bed when you cannot sleep. This is a good idea for a few minutes, but if you find that after 10–20 minutes you're still awake and your mind is active or you're feeling worried, then it is a good idea to get out of bed. Finding a quiet space to meditate, listen to some soothing music or do something that relaxes you can help to prepare both your mind and body for sleep. Once you feel tired again, you can try going back to bed.

Counting sheep is an option; however, the first thing you would need to do is imagine the sheep, which takes your mind into an active phase and makes it harder for you to fall asleep! Focusing your attention on your breathing and counting each in-breath and out-breath is a far more effective option.

Try this simple breathing meditation to help you fall asleep:

- Lying in your bed, find a comfortable position and gently bring your attention to your breathing. Don't try to change how you are breathing; just spend a moment noticing each in-breath and each out-breath.
- When you are ready, take a deeper breath in, hold your breath for a second, and then slowly breathe out (this is breath one).
- Repeat this for up to ten breaths – breathing in, holding the breath, and then slowly breathing out.

- Keep counting the breaths, from one to ten and then back to one again, until you fall asleep.

Sleep myth 3: Napping stops you from sleeping at night

Napping is fine and can give you a 'second wind' at times in the day when you feel fatigued. Your body's circadian rhythm has its ups and downs throughout the day, so there will be times when you feel more tired. In a typical 9–5 work day, this often happens after lunch. If your sleep is being disrupted because you're working long shifts, sleeping poorly due to worry or anxiety, managing childcare or home-schooling, or self-isolating, scheduling in a power nap can help to boost your energy.

A power nap is anything between 10–30 minutes, and it gives the mind and body time to recharge. It's like charging your smartphone for five minutes when it's running out of battery and you need to make an important call – you can boost the battery just enough for your call, until you have the opportunity to charge it fully.

Sleep myth 4: Snoring may be annoying, but it's not dangerous

Snoring is definitely irritating for the partner whose sleep is affected by it, and when we find ourselves spending more time at home together, this irritation may grow. However, snoring can also be a sign of sleep apnoea: a disorder where the breathing stops momentarily before suddenly starting again. If snoring is an issue for you or your partner, seek medical advice.

Sleep myth 5: During sleep, your brain rests

During sleep, the body rests, not the brain. The brain is always active. Sleeping gives the brain opportunities to restore and repair, preparing you to be alert and functioning well the next day. The brain has to remain active to control your heart and lungs, as well as other functions of your body.

Tips for Sleeping Well During Difficult Times

Good sleep hygiene involves pre-bedtime routines and consistent wake times. Children usually have a bedtime routine – perhaps a bath, a bedtime story, maybe a warm drink of milk – and adults can find a routine equally helpful.

The idea of good sleep hygiene is to create a pause between our daytime routines and our sleep routines, which helps to prepare both our mind and body for bed.

Here are my top sleep hygiene tips for a better night's sleep:

- Avoid fatty foods before bedtime. The digestive system has to work hard to digest the fat, which can lead to heartburn.
- Avoid alcohol and caffeine. Any chemical substance that disrupts sleep patterns and cycles should be avoided before sleep. Instead, try a relaxing herbal drink, such as chamomile tea.
- Turn off your technology. The blue light emitted by technology fools the brain into thinking it is still daytime. Turn off notifications, the TV and social media an hour

before going to bed, and charge your devices in a different room than your bedroom.

- Set a bedtime routine, to include time and space for relaxing and switching off. Perhaps spend time reading, have a bath, or do some light yoga or meditation. You may like to try my **seven-minute breathing meditation as part of your pre-sleep routine** at TeachMindfulnessOnline.com/book.

- Avoid strenuous exercise. Regular exercise can support better sleep; however, high-impact exercise is not recommended just before bedtime. Light yoga or gentle stretches an hour before sleeping can prepare both your mind and body for sleep.

- Disengage with the news and social media as the stories and updates can increase anxiety. Limit yourself to one reliable source of news, and unfollow negative or sensationalised media sources.

- Make your bedroom a space for sleeping. Take out the technology, invest in a good quality mattress, keep the temperature a little cool, use clean sheets and bedding, put up blackout curtains or blinds, and declutter the room, making it a place of calm and serenity.

- Try soothing essential oils, in a pre-sleep bath or as a drop of oil near your pillow. Lavender is thought to aid sleep.

Remember:

- High-quality sleep is essential for overall health and wellbeing. Aiming for 7–9 hours of sleep per night (more for children and young adults) can help you to cope during challenging times.

- A bedtime routine that works with your lifestyle, work and family commitments will help you to prepare your mind and body for sleep.
- Resist the urge to check the news or social media before you go to bed. Replace with a mindful practice such as meditation, or perhaps read a calming book. Your bedroom is for sleeping and recharging your energy, so try to create a calming space for you to rest.

About Jane Bozier

Jane is a registered mental health nurse with 35 years' experience. She has a master's degree in mindfulness and has been practising and teaching mindfulness for 10 years. She is based in Luton, Bedfordshire, UK.

6

Mindfulness in the Presence of Traumatic Memories

Amy Malloy

When times feel difficult, it can be very tempting to run away and pretend they aren't happening. Or you may desperately go in circles to fix things, to no avail. These are very normal responses to stressful situations. Mindfulness is so effective and attractive because it helps us notice what is happening in the present and, using patience, non-judgement and compassion, learn to cope with both the ups and downs of life with greater ease. In short, if something difficult happens, it doesn't have to feel so difficult. Mindfulness helps us notice it, accept it and move on.

However, what if the present moment is too unbearable to experience directly, so blocking it out isn't habit, it's survival? Some survivors of traumatic events experience this every day, posing significant challenges for emotional, social and physical interaction. When you then face difficult times as well, it may feel like many of the resources available don't work for you.

While much evidence exists around the effectiveness of mindfulness for trauma recovery, here I look at the reality in practice when the usual constants around you feel unsteady. This chapter explores the benefits and challenges of mindfulness meditation with traumatic memories, proposing steps to keep your practice safe and restorative, while helping you practise on your own terms.

Fight/Flight/Freeze and the Post-traumatic Response

A business studies tutor at school once said that business had become very complicated, and that sometimes you needed to go back to the basics of selling lemonade at the side of the road in order to understand a business concept.

The same approach is useful here, too. When we are talking about any response to stressful times, we are really referring to our survival instinct. So let's go back to when survive was all we did: back to the caves.

Up to around 70,000 years ago, we lived in our emotional brain, the oldest part in evolution and the first to develop as babies. Over time, we have evolved more rational thought, but then it was simply us versus predator, in the moment. If a sabre-toothed tiger approached our cave, our brains gave our bodies three choices: fight the tiger, run away or play dead. Fight, flight or freeze.

Of the two branches of the nervous system, the one controlling this response is the autonomic nervous system, which itself has two branches: sympathetic (fight or flight) and parasympathetic (rest and digest).

Here's what happened in our caveman's body. The sympathetic branch of the nervous system sprang into action and prompted the stress hormones adrenaline and cortisol to be released. They raised our heart rate, sharpened our vision, hunched our shoulders and bunched up our hips ready to either run or punch and kick. Survival of the fittest. Man versus beast. Sometimes, the body would shut down to play dead until it was over (dissociating from the threat).

Once the threat had passed, the parasympathetic nervous system took over to calm us down. Releasing oxytocin, the 'love hormone', the breath and heart rate slowed and the muscles relaxed, telling the body it was now safe to rest, to digest food and to procreate. This response has remained in us to this day, even after our brains have evolved to be capable of more rational and strategic thought.

Generally, our memory function in the brain kicks in to let us know that the threat has passed. The experience then becomes integrated into our working memory: our mind archives the event, replays and reworks it, and integrates it into the past, telling our nervous system that the threat has passed.

Sometimes a threatening event feels too distressing for the memory to integrate it. We keep the threat alive as if it were in the present moment, to stop us forgetting the danger. This is what is called a *post-traumatic response*, and it can relate to both physical and emotional threats. This is a completely normal human response to an abnormal situation.

Mindfulness in Challenging Times, alongside Traumatic Memories

Mindfulness is considered a cornerstone of healing practices for post-traumatic responses. It encourages growth of the prefrontal cortex (the rational brain, which evolved later) to help us make sense of our experiences, including emotional regulation and facilitating empathy and trust in ourselves and in others. It helps us tell the difference between habitual spiralling thoughts and real, present-moment sensations. From a trauma-recovery perspective, it can teach the mind (and the nervous system) that physical sensations are impermanent and ultimately safe to experience.

Mindfulness teaches us to meet good and bad experiences equally. We are encouraged to sit with and even lean into challenges, debunk the narrative around the suffering challenges creates, and accept the situation as it is. We work on identifying a pause before responding, noticing what's going on and responding carefully rather than reacting impulsively. However, if you have unsettled traumatic memories, being asked to lean into difficult sensations could simply be too much for your nervous system to handle, so you need to approach your mindfulness practice with more flexibility and care.

If a memory of a traumatic event remains unsettled, our brain bypasses the more rational prefrontal cortex (which makes that pause possible), and instead triggers a fight, flight or freeze response to a much less serious event that in some way reminds the body of the original threat. Dissociating – essentially, checking out until it's over – is common. This certainly doesn't mean that you're 'bad' at mindfulness – there is no being bad at mindfulness. A post-traumatic response is a completely normal human response to an abnormal situation. Remember, it is our body's way of stopping us from forgetting the distressing situation, so we don't do it again.

The result can often be a constant feeling of not being safe in one's own body or mind. Rather than looking inwards and being present, we seek to do anything but.

While mindfulness is a really supportive practice for traumatic memories during times of challenge, we need to practise flexibly to keep within our window of tolerance – the boundaries within which you are able to respond to your everyday experiences without difficulty. This window might be smaller than it has been for you previously, but in time and with care it can widen again.

Modifications for Practising Mindfulness with Trauma

My personal experience of past trauma left me with a strong resistance to being told what to do. If I acquiesced, I was back to feeling small, like a child, with all the vulnerable feelings I associated with that. I also struggled (and still do) with making decisions, for fear of making the wrong choice. Mindfulness has been a major part of my personal mental health recovery, along with yoga. Working through this experience in adult life, I learned firstly that I have a choice and agency over my actions, and secondly that whatever I choose is the right decision for me at that moment.

I have found the following strategies helpful, which have also informed my teaching of both yoga and mindfulness, regardless of who is in the class. You never know what battles people are facing and, quite simply, everyone deserves to feel in charge of their own experience. Mindfulness is accessible for all – simply do what works for you.

Keep your eyes open

Traditionally, we are invited to close our eyes to focus on our body and breath. It is a beautiful practice and one that I personally find really peaceful. But this may not feel right for you, so try keeping your eyes either open with a softened gaze, or fully open if this feels more comfortable.

Move if you want to

Meditation is usually practised sitting or lying still. However, sometimes this isn't comfortable. If stillness feels overwhelming, try coming into some gentle movement while you focus on your breath. Perhaps a gentle sway from side to side, or floating your arms up as you inhale and down as you exhale. Whenever you feel comfortable, slow down a bit. You can find stillness in your own time.

Keep it short, and be gentle with body scan meditations

As mentioned earlier, the fight/flight response bypasses your conscious brain. It sends signals from the nervous system straight to the body (for speed). This means much of the memory of the trauma is held in your body. Sometimes, focusing too closely on parts of the body can activate flashbacks and overwhelming responses if the traumatic memory is unresolved. It is safer to stick to focusing on how your inhale and exhale feel, rather than specifically on sensations around the body. If you would like to try a body scan, then go for a progressive muscle relaxation, where you tense and release each bit of your body in turn. Keep meditations shorter than you might normally, too.

Pick the posture that suits you

You may see lots of pictures of people meditating with legs crossed or bent around their head. It really doesn't matter how you sit when you practise mindfulness. If you feel more comfortable standing up, kneeling or lying down, then do just that. Find the posture that works for you, knowing that you can move whenever you need to. You may also like to place a blanket over yourself if you're lying down.

Practise in a comforting space, with external senses to ground you

Holding a comforting object, or a piece of tissue with a scent that you know comforts you, can be a really helpful way to keep you grounded in the present moment during your meditation. Carefully selected music can also be a helpful point of focus, as is keeping one hand resting on the ground throughout.

Stay within your window of tolerance

When we're living with traumatic memories, our window of tolerance for stress greatly reduces. It doesn't take much to become hyper-aroused (where we spring into panic) or hypo-aroused (where we shut down and dissociate from what is happening). All of these modifications can help you stay within your window of tolerance and give you a way back to the present reality if you feel you may be slipping.

Grounding and Supportive Trauma-aware Meditations

If you are living with post-traumatic stress, your practice needs a balance between keeping you grounded in the present, while also gently reintegrating the memory so you can view it from afar rather than relive it.

Grounding (a three-minute meditation): The 5-4-3-2-1

This is a lovely short practice that you can do anywhere if you start to feel a little overwhelmed by your mind, or feel you may dissociate.

1. Sit or stand comfortably, with your eyes open.
2. Notice five things around you that you can see. Label them and move on.
3. Close or soften the eyes. Notice four things you can hear, then three things you can feel. Label them and move on.
4. Notice two things you can smell, then one thing you can taste. Label them and move on.

Gently restoring (a ten-minute meditation): Coherent breathing

Coherent breathing is the practice of breathing slowly and deeply (usually about five to six breaths per minute) to synchronise your breath and heart rate, evoking calm. You can actively tell the nervous system you are safe again by steadying your breath and activating the calming vagus nerve, thus gently increasing your window of tolerance. Listen to the track at TeachMindfulnessOnline.com/book to try this out.

Remember:

- When you have experienced trauma in your past, you may not find it feels safe to focus on internal anchors in the body. You may wish to leave the inner world well alone. When we are stuck in fight or flight mode, we lack the space to notice our reactions – and they would be too painful if we could.

- Handled skilfully on your terms, mindfulness is a really powerful tool to support post-traumatic growth. Opening yourself up safely to your inner experience makes it possible to take back control and agency over your body and your mind so you feel safe again.
- It's really important that you take this agency back slowly, with the support of a professional trauma therapist, and by keeping your mindfulness practice flexible, on your terms and within your window of tolerance. In this way, your mindfulness practice can be accessible, safe and ultimately healing.

About Amy Malloy

Amy is the founder of social enterprise No More Shoulds, with the mission to provide simple access to yoga, mindfulness and other healing practices for better mental health. She's based in the Oxfordshire Cotswolds, UK.

www.nomoreshoulds.com

Consultant and endorsement

Ewen Sim (MSc Psychological Trauma and trauma-informed mindfulness specialist for Lancashire Constabulary) provided an additional review of this chapter.

7

Being Mindful with Grief

Linda Shalloe

Grief is one of the facets of life that is always challenging. We experience grief when we are coping with a loss or a difficult change in our lives.

This could be the loss of a loved one, such as a family member, a partner, a friend or a pet; it could be a broken relationship, a diagnosis of an illness or fear for the future; it could be the loss of a home or a job – they all cause grief in different ways.

You may start to grieve for someone before they die, maybe because of a difficult relationship that couldn't be reconciled due to terminal illness or a life-changing incident.

You may experience grief when a pandemic hits globally, as with the coronavirus pandemic: we grieve for our world, our communities, our close ones and indeed ourselves. This is *transitional grief*: a growing awareness that things are changing, and feelings of grief and sadness arise because of the many losses involved – not only the loss of human life, but also the loss of beliefs, identities and lifestyles.

Whatever the change, we have an internal realisation that life will never be the same again after the event; that this loss or change, whether major or minor, will alter our lives or our pathways forever.

How Do We Deal with Grief Mindfully?

"The pain I feel now is the happiness I had before." C.S. Lewis

No matter what we are grieving for, we need to open a space in our hearts gently, with kindness and compassion. We need to let go of judgement and have patience, as we hold our own hands and our own hearts and create a space of hope.

When you experience grief, don't try to do too much. Don't expect too much of yourself, and remind yourself that although life might still be moving normally around you, it is not the same for you. Learn to care for yourself gently.

There are different phases in grief – denial, anger, bargaining, depression, acceptance – which you can find out more about online if you wish. When you allow yourself to feel every emotion in each of these five phases, whatever emotion is present, take the time to acknowledge that you are experiencing an emotion you have never felt in this way before, and every loss you experience will be different.

You may move from one of these phases to another for some time. They come in no particular order. Do your best to be kind to yourself when each phase is present, recognising that each phase needs time and is helping you in the healing process as you arrive at the phase of acceptance.

We all grieve differently, and you will have many ups and downs – many devastating moments of sadness, hurt, pain, hopelessness and loss, but also uplifting moments of joy, laughter, compassion, hope and love. You can use mindfulness no matter what your grief is; the techniques will help you process all your emotions, helping you to connect with yourself in truth and with thoughtfulness.

Using Self-care with Grief

When my dad passed away to cancer at the age of 68, all phases of grief paid a visit. The most difficult ones for me were anger, guilt and acceptance. I kept all the pain alive in my thoughts and in my feelings: all the anger towards his medical team, and the anger against his cancer, overwhelmed me, as well as the guilt that I did not do enough to save him, to help him live longer. Although it was all out of my control, my thoughts played tricks, making me believe things that were not true.

To help myself, I chose kindness. I started to work with myself the very same way I would a client, a family member or friend who was grieving, by using a programme of self-care. I focused on myself and nourished my anguish, pain and loss. I spent time with people I loved and distanced myself from people I found difficult. I needed to be me, with no rushing, no judging and no expectations as I looked for comfort from the inside.

Being mindful with grief and participating in the programme of self-care encouraged self-awareness. As a teacher and practitioner of mindfulness meditation, I know that mindfulness can be as simple as taking time to pay attention to your breath, or as complex as aiming to calm the nervous system, focus the mind, and become aware of the body, the breath, the present moment and ultimately the stillness within us and around us. Regardless of your particular methods of mindfulness and self-care, the key is individualising it to your life and your needs.

Crafting a Programme of Self-care

Ask yourself these questions:

- What do I need to do right now to help myself feel better?
- What are the most important aspects of my life?
- What helps me stay connected to what is important?
- What helps me feel content?

By keeping it simple, your answers will come.

These were my answers:

- Using my breath (you may like to try my breathing in comfort meditation: visit: TeachMindfulnessOnline.com/book)
- Wrapping myself in a warm blanket and feeling its comfort
- Listening to guided meditations
- Spending time in nature

- Having my favourite food and drinks
- Listening to music, and being creative
- Spending time with people who care
- Talking or writing about anything that came to mind, and writing poetry (you may like to listen to my poem called 'Hello Grief': visit TeachMindfulnessOnline.com/book)
- Cultivating gratitude (see Chapter 12 for more on gratitude)
- Listening to someone else's story
- Creating a sleep/rest plan
- Seeing a bereavement/grief counsellor

When you decide on what can help you, make time for it. Create a timetable of self-care for yourself, even if you have returned to your 'normal daily life'. No matter how busy your schedule or difficult your life is, you can still find moments to practise self-care. Know that every day will be different, so check in with yourself often throughout your day, listen to what you need and be your own best friend.

Consider setting an alarm hourly to check in with yourself to see how you're doing. Acknowledge both difficult and easy moments, and realise they will pass.

Treat yourself with care, love and kindness, whatever the emotion you are feeling, with no judgement:

- **What is your emotion at this time?** Stop and notice how you feel (sad, overwhelmed, angry, numb, hurt, anxious, joyful, relaxed?).

- **Acknowledge your emotion.** Are you ok with it? Would you like to feel differently?

- **What mindfulness technique or wellbeing activity can you do in this moment to help yourself feel better?** Know that you can go back to the list you created with your self-care programme. Tweak and enhance it as often as you wish.

- **Consider your mood after using mindfulness and following your self-care programme.** Do you feel better, worse or the same?

As with the five phases of grief, there is no set plan; adjust and tweak your own self-care programme as you need to. The pace at which you grieve and how you grieve your loss is as unique as you are: no two people will grieve the same.

Moving towards Acceptance

It helped me to speak to my dad quietly and then listen, as I remember his voice and laughter. When I'm with others now, I speak about him openly; I laugh and smile when I remember the good times we had, and I cry whenever I need to. I celebrate his life as I have grieved his death.

My mind is quieter, my anger has dissipated, my guilt has eased and clarity has taken their place. Clarity arrived when my soul whispered one day, "How many times did your dad die?" I can honestly say it jolted me! When I was able, I whispered back, "Once; he died once." Then the whisper came, "How many times have you made him die?" I whispered back, "So many times."

In that moment I let my dad rest, and my mind rested too, in the realisation that I couldn't change what had already happened. No matter how many times I wanted it to be different, and no matter how angry I felt, it didn't change what I wanted to change.

In my grief, I needed to meander just like a river – always moving, even though the flow may be slowed or blocked. I also moved slowly and gently, mindfully and compassionately, to the phase of acceptance.

I wish you well; I wish you kindness, gentleness and compassion in your challenges of life, no matter what your grief.

Remember:

- Understand that grief has many phases and no time limit.
- There is no rulebook on grief; there is no right or wrong way to grieve.
- Give yourself time and a programme of self-care to nurture and soothe yourself.

About Linda Shalloe

Based in the Republic of Ireland, Linda has been a mindfulness and holistic therapist practitioner for over 15 years. She helps people to focus on their wellbeing, encouraging them to tap into their inner resources to live a happier, healthier and more fulfilling life.

www.lindashalloe.com

8

A Mindful Approach to Managing Your Media Consumption

Annemarie Wiegand

"I am not afraid of storms, for I am learning how to sail my ship."
Louisa May Alcott

This quote feels very fitting as we reflect on the uncertain and unsettling times we have found ourselves in during the coronavirus crisis of 2020. Dark thunder clouds have rolled in, hovering over our skies as we move forward into uncharted waters, individually as well as collectively, across our communities, our countries and the world.

With this storm, and often during other difficult times we may face in our lives, it's worth remembering that the Chinese word for 'crisis' is composed of two characters – one represents danger, and the other represents opportunity. The way that we consume media and connect using technology has evolved during this crisis. Although excess media consumption can be detrimental, when we are open to learning how to navigate it differently we can begin to see it as a new opportunity for connection and mindfulness.

The Benefits and Drawbacks of Instant-access Media

During challenging times (both virus and non-virus related), social media and communication technology are lifelines that keep us connected to our workplaces, friends and family, and to reports of events unfolding around the world.

It has been incredibly uplifting to see the amazing responses and reactions of people all over the world during the recent crisis period. From 24-hour access to news and information – as well as opportunities to connect through apps and services such as FaceTime, Facebook Live, Instagram, TikTok, Zoom and Houseparty – this period of crisis has encouraged us to embrace technology and media in all its forms in a different and more engaging way than we may have done in the past. Being able to video call, keep regular contact on WhatsApp and send videos of my 18-month-old daughter's playful antics to my friends and family (including my 90-year-old grandmother who, yes, is active on Facebook) has been a beacon of light and provided many giggles for us all during these isolating and often lonely times.

However, as we look to these ubiquitous media channels for information, entertainment, distraction or connection, we must do so while being conscious of how much time we are spending on them, what purpose they are serving, and what impact they are having on our mental health.

While writing this chapter, I asked a group of friends about their media consumption during these challenging times. Some of their responses included:

- "I started YouTube yoga and exercise classes, which are keeping me active and sane."
- "I found myself listening to the news all day."
- "I had the TV on from morning to evening to hear the latest news. I found myself wanting to know every detail happening here and across the UK, Europe, the US and the world. It was consuming me, and I started to feel short-tempered with myself and my family, getting headaches and generally feeling rubbish."
- "I found I had my phone in my hand 24/7 looking at the news and WhatsApp messages from family, friends, teachers and parent groups – it was bombarding and endless."
- "I've begun to limit my news updates to once a day and have started to leave my phone upstairs during the day so I am more present with my family and the activities I am doing."

I'm sure these are common responses and insights. Our consumption of media doesn't define us, but unconsciously consuming media may have lasting negative impacts.

Statista reported in March 2020 that people spend an average of 463 minutes, or over 7.5 <u>hours, per day with media</u>. What's wrong with that? A moderate amount of media consumption is fine, but too much time on your device can lead to bad habits forming.

There is growing science around this topic. Research has shown that getting social media notifications from our smartphones is like carrying around little dopamine stimulators in our pockets. Upon receiving a notification, the brain sends a chemical message (dopamine) along our reward pathway, which makes us feel good. This can become addictive, so we check our devices constantly. (Trevor Haynes summarised the latest research very effectively in 2018 in a Harvard University blog article.)

Recent research (as explained in the TED-Ed video, '5 Ways Social Media is Changing Your Brain Right Now') has found that, over time, excess social media use can make us bad at multitasking. Although you might think the opposite, research has shown that excess social media usage impacts your brain by making it harder for you to commit information to memory. Furthermore, social media can become a psychological addiction through broken reward pathways in our brains. Social media provides immediate rewards in the form of attention from your network for minimal effort. This can cause the brain to rewire itself, making you desire likes, retweets and emoji applause, and respond instantaneously to notifications. Five to 10 per cent of internet users are psychologically addicted and can't control how much time they spend online. Brain scans show a clear change in the regions of the brain that control emotions, attention and decision-making.

Introducing a Mindful Approach to Managing Your Media Consumption

The ways in which we consume media and utilise communication technology provide us with an opportunity to connect mindfully with others, while avoiding excess media. Here is where the magic of living and practising mindfulness regularly can help. By adopting a mindset of optimism and curiosity, we can learn how to navigate our ship (ourselves) and be open to considering mindfulness in relation to our media consumption. Mindfulness allows us to truly experience the current moment and integrate that awareness into our everyday life and activities.

Mindfulness can help us to STOP. This simple four-step exercise helps you to press the pause button before mindlessly picking up your device, and it has the potential to bring about significant changes in your habits, feelings and behaviours.

S = Stop
Stop what you are doing. Press the pause button on your thoughts and actions.

T = Take a Breath
Take a few deep breaths to centre yourself and bring yourself fully into the present moment.

O = Observe
Observe what is going on with your:
- **Body:** What physical sensations are you aware of (touch, sight, hearing, taste, smell)?
- **Emotions:** What are you feeling right now?
- **Mind:** What assumptions are you making about your feelings? What is the story you're telling yourself about why you are having them?

P = Proceed
Proceed with whatever you were doing, making a conscious, intentional choice to incorporate what you just learned.

Let's try applying the STOP approach with this social media mindfulness practice.

S = Stop
- Sit comfortably in an alert and ready posture.
- Roll your shoulders, take a few breaths, and bring awareness to your physical and emotional state in this particular moment.
- Now, open your computer or click on your phone.

T = Take
- Before you open your favourite social media or news site, consider your intentions and expectations. As you focus on the icon, notice the experiences you have in your mind and body.

O = Observe
- Why are you about to check this site?
- What are you hoping to see or not see?
- How are you going to respond to the different kinds of updates you encounter?
- By checking your device, are you interested in connecting or in disconnecting and distracting?
- Close your eyes and focus on your emotional state for three breaths.

P = Proceed
- Opening your eyes, look at the first news item, status update or photo, and then sit back and close your eyes again.
- Notice your response, your emotion. Is it excitement? Boredom? Jealousy? Regret? Fear?

- How do you experience this emotion in your mind and body? Do you feel you want to read on, to click a response, to share yourself, or something else?
- Wait for a breath or two for the sensations and emotions to fade, or focus on your breath, body or surrounding sounds.
- Try this practice for three or five minutes daily, ideally over seven days, depending on your time and your practice.

I also share a short guided audio practice to guide you through using the STOP approach to mindfully manage your media consumption (visit TeachMindfulnessOnline.com/book).

How has that made you feel?

Taking the time to practise mindful media consumption is an investment in **YOU**: the most important person there is. I would encourage you to make this investment to help you discover how your media consumption makes you feel and how to use it more mindfully.

Bringing awareness to this activity will make you more conscious of the emotions and feelings you are inviting into your day and your mind. Doing this regularly, with kindness and openness to yourself, can unlock your potential to make better, more mindful decisions about how you engage with and consume media. It can alert you to times when you may be going into excess.

Lastly, remember that during times of crisis, the rational mind doesn't always come to the fore. We are humans, with feelings, emotions, wishes and desires. Mindfulness requires us to take one step at a time. Don't worry when you slip up, as I have done many times.

The modern science of media and its presence in our lives is complex and often has a significant influence over our basic human emotions. So, be kind to yourself and allow yourself time to mindfully connect with media.

Remember:

- Examine your media consumption, how your time is being spent, and what purpose it is serving you.
- Apply the STOP approach when you use your device.
- Engage with these new ways of making technology serve you in order to foster connected wellness.

About Annemarie Wiegand

Annemarie is an HR professional, a mindfulness teacher and a mother. Her YouTube channel, 'The Mindful Mammy', is dedicated to sharing and experiencing the simplicity and power of mindful meditations that help parents to live mindfully, and feel well and calm. She lives in Dubai, UAE.

YouTube: The Mindful Mammy

PART 2
PRACTISING SELF-CARE, COMPASSION AND KINDNESS

9

Mindful Yoga

Jamila Knopp

When I started practising yoga in my early twenties, I felt drawn to it for the physical aspects of improving flexibility and strength. But then, to my surprise, I noticed that yoga was offering me much more. I felt calmer and more connected with myself after each practice. It was like coming home to myself. I saw for myself that yoga works on much more than just the physical level. And little did I know that, ten years later, I would study to be a yoga teacher and that it would save me from burnout in my late thirties.

In challenging times, we are often more stressed then we realise. Whereas small amounts of stress can be beneficial in motivating us to get a task done, chronic or long-term stress can be very detrimental. It is, therefore, essential that we recognise when we are stressed and what causes us stress so that we can start making changes.

Mindful yoga offers an opportunity to pause and to bring conscious attention to the present moment. This conscious attention will also extend into your everyday life. Anyone can practise mindful yoga, no matter your age or flexibility. It is especially useful for people who find it challenging to do mindfulness practices while sitting or lying still. Mindful yoga is a combination of movement and stillness.

What is Yoga?

"Yoga is the journey of the self, through the self, to the self." *The Bhagavad Gita*

Yoga is an ancient practice from India, and the word 'yoga' means union – a union of the individual with the universe, with nature, with others and with oneself. This union contributes to a life filled with peace, contentment and a positive attitude.

Yoga is more than just a physical practice: it is for the body, mind and spirit. Yoga helps you to feel balanced and whole.

What is Mindful Yoga?

With mindfulness, we practise awareness and learn to slow down. In mindful yoga, we focus more on the here and now and learn to stay present in our practice. We move slowly and deliberately, and there are moments of stillness for reflection. Our attention is single-focused, on only one thing at a time. We observe and focus on our body, our breath, our thoughts, any sounds or how we feel. You can bring these principles to any yoga practice to make it a mindful yoga practice.

Mindful yoga helps us manage stress and is beneficial for our body, mind and emotions. The antidote to toxic stress is mindful awareness. To be mindful is to be aware and awake with kindness, curiosity and acceptance.

Breathing

One way we can explore mindfulness is through our breathing. Both mindful yoga and calming breathing can switch the body from operating from the sympathetic nervous system (being stressed) to the parasympathetic nervous system (being relaxed).

Our breath is a barometer for our overall physical and mental state, and it's also the foundation of mindfulness. Practising mindful breathing is key to calming the body and mind.

In yoga, breathing techniques are called *pranayama*. My favourite type of pranayama is alternate nostril breathing.

There are many great reasons to practise this breathing technique daily, and here are a few of its benefits:

- Improves focus and clarity
- Calms your mind and emotions
- Improves sleep
- Is an excellent preparation for meditation
- Soothes your nervous system
- Enhances rest and relaxation

Even after only two minutes of alternate nostril breathing, you may notice a difference in how you feel.

How to do mindful alternate nostril breathing

As best as you can, stay focused on your breathing. When your mind wanders, guide it back kindly to your breath.

Close your eyes or keep them open with a gentle gaze. Sit comfortably with your shoulders at ease and bring your right hand up to your nose. Close off the right nostril with your thumb and inhale through the left nostril fully. At the end of that inhalation, close off the left nostril with your ring finger and then release the right nostril and exhale.

Next, inhale deeply through the right nostril, close it off and then release the left nostril as you exhale completely through it. Then inhale deeply through the left, repeating the cycle. Let the breath flow from side to side.

Do this as many times as you like, being sure to exhale through the left nostril to complete your last cycle.

Once you get used to doing this breathing exercise, you can use the count of *4–12–8*. Inhale to the count of 4, hold your breath to the count of 12 and exhale to the count of 8.

I share a short guided audio practice to guide you through alternate nostril breathing
(visit TeachMindfulnessOnline.com/book).

When is a Good Time to Practise Yoga?

A great time to practise is in the morning after getting up, when your mind is naturally calmer. Or you might like to have a short practice while taking a break from work or chores. Another good time is after work as an in-between time for yourself, when you can let go of your day before you connect with your loved ones.

It's easier to stick to your practice and to create a new habit of making this part of your day when you always practise at the same time. You can connect the practice with something else that you do daily, such as before eating breakfast, after your shower, after you get home or before bedtime.

Whatever your situation, remember that it takes patience and regular daily mindfulness practice to create change.

Tips for Mindful Yoga Practice

1. Try setting your intention before you start your practice, which will help to focus and motivate you. Think of a small intention: "Today, I will do my best and let go of any expectations", or "Today, I will bring kindness to my practice."
2. Bring the attitudes of kindness, non-judgement, openness and curiosity to your practice.
3. Have patience with yourself and your practice. If you lose concentration or don't feel the stretch much, that is okay and normal. Just be aware of your experience as it is.
4. If your mind wanders, try not to judge yourself. As soon as you notice this, just guide your attention kindly back to the mindful yoga. The mind-wandering is part of your practice.
5. You doing your practice is enough and perfect as it is. It doesn't need to be any other way. How does it feel when you let go of any expectations? Just allow your practice to

be as it is. Mindful yoga is more about 'being' than 'doing'.

How to Practise Mindful Yoga

"In this moment, there is plenty of time. In this moment, you are precisely as you should be. In this moment, there is infinite possibility." Victoria Moran

To practise mindful yoga, focus on your breath and body sensations as best as you can. Try and practise with kindness. It is not about pushing yourself but rather to cultivate awareness of breath and body.

Notice any thoughts or emotions as you move and stretch. Just go at your own pace, and if a pose doesn't feel right, then don't hold it. Be extra careful if you are recovering from an injury. Listen to your body, practise at your own speed and adjust the poses when you need to. If your mind wanders, that's okay; just kindly guide it back to focus on your practice without judging or criticising yourself.

You can listen to my guided audio track of a short practice (visit TeachMindfulnessOnline.com/book), or you can follow this practice here.

Begin by standing in Mountain Pose, with your feet hip-width apart and your knees soft and relaxed. Keep your back straight. Get a sense of yourself standing firmly on the ground. Close your eyes for a moment and take a few deep breaths. As you inhale, get a sense of lengthening up and, as you exhale, imagine breathing out down into your feet, connecting with the ground. Tune into your body and become aware of your whole body.

Breathe in, lifting your arms slowly until they are above your head. Have your palms facing each other, and your arms about shoulder-width apart. Looking forward, on an exhale, move your arms and upper body to the right, keeping both feet firmly on the ground. Hold this gentle stretch for a breath or two. Keep your breathing easy.

On an inhale, move up to the middle and, on the exhale, move over to the left side. Hold this stretch for a breath or two and, when you are ready, breathe in and move back to the centre, and then move your arms down slowly to your sides.

For the next pose, keep your knees soft and slightly bent. When you inhale, lift your arms up and then, on the exhale, slowly bend forward from your hips, moving your torso and head as one unit. Then just gently rest in the standing forward bend for a moment.

Then, when you are ready, touch the ground with your hands, step back with your right leg and drop the right knee to the ground, with your hands on the ground under your shoulders. Continue to hold this lunge for a moment. Then step forward into a standing forward bend and step back with your left leg and drop the left knee, holding this lunge for a moment. Then, lift the left knee and step back with your right foot into Plank Pose. Try and hold this pose for a moment or, if this is too much, drop your knees down to the floor.

Next is the Cat and Cow Pose. Begin with your hands and knees on the floor, with your knees below your hips and your hands below your shoulders. Try and do these postures with your eyes closed. Exhale as you slowly tuck your chin towards your chest, lift your mid-back towards the ceiling and scoop your tailbone under like a scared cat. Inhale as you drop your belly and lift your gaze and your tail bone into Cow Pose.

Do at least four rounds of Cat and Cow Pose, then sit back on your heels and lower your forehead to rest on the ground. Keep your knees apart and rest your arms by the sides of your body, with the palms facing up. If you prefer, stretch your arms forward. Rest in this Child Pose for a moment. Allow your back to relax completely. Notice your breathing and how your belly moves against your legs when you inhale. With each exhale, welcome a sense of letting go.

When you are ready, move up onto your hands and knees again, tuck your toes under and lift your hips into an upside-down V: Downward-Facing Dog Pose. Your legs are straight, and your heels move towards the floor. Try and walk a little on the spot slowly by bending one knee at a time without lifting your feet of the ground. Do this gently and slowly, and then hold the pose for a moment.

Now bend your knees and move down onto your belly, keeping your hands where they are by the side of your shoulders. Breathe in and let go as you exhale.

And then move into Cobra Pose on the next inhale, lifting your head and chest slowly and carefully. Only move up as high as you are comfortable with in your lower back. Keep your shoulders down. Take a breath and then, on the exhale, move down again.

And now comes a great pose: Shavasana, resting on your back. Moving slowly, put on a jacket, or grab a blanket to make sure that you will be warm. Lie on your back, with your palms facing up, allowing your feet to fall outwards to the sides. Slowly roll your head from side to side two or three times to release your neck. Then take three deep breaths, breathing in deeply and out fully.

Do a short body scan, taking your awareness from your feet up to your head (refer to Chapter 4 for more on the body scan – I also include a short body scan in my guided audio track for this mindful yoga practice).

As your practice comes to an end, give yourself credit for having spent this time deeply nourishing yourself. Allow the benefits of this practice to expand into every aspect of your life.

Remember:

- Slowing down with mindful yoga and feeling its restorative power works wonders for your health and wellbeing. It helps you to manage stress and is beneficial for your body, mind and emotions.
- With mindful yoga, we focus on the here and now and learn to stay present in our practice. We move slowly and deliberately, and there are moments of stillness for reflection.
- Your body is brilliant and can heal itself from stress. Mindful yoga, combined with regular walking and the other calming mindfulness practices described in this book, can do you a lot of good. Try to stay positive, even in challenging times. Be aware of your thoughts. A positive attitude is fundamental to helping you get through a stressful period with more ease.

"You have a treasure within you that is infinitely greater than anything the world can offer." Eckhart Tolle

About Jamila Knopp

Jamila lives in New Zealand. She is a mindfulness and yoga teacher as well as an Ayurveda practitioner. Jamila's clients often say that she teaches in a kind, calm and caring way.

www.turningpointnz.com

10

Mindful Eating

Lucie Kysučanová

Food forms a major part of our daily lives, whether or not we're experiencing challenging times. Perhaps, during lockdown, you have been enjoying baking and trying new recipes. Food is necessary for our survival, but it is also something most people enjoy. Therefore, practising mindful eating provides a great opportunity for us to bring a more mindful approach to something we would do anyway.

Mindful eating can bring many benefits, especially during challenging times. Regular mindful eating practice has been shown to help with different eating disorders and raise positive body image. It helps to create healthy eating habits and change unhealthy beliefs about food, and it can even help you learn to connect with your body in order to better understand what it needs to stay well, joyful and full of energy.

Considering Your Relationship with Food

Our perception of food and the customs we associate with our meals vary with each individual and can hold different meanings. For some, food is both the first and the last thing we experience every day, for some it is something that requires forward planning, and for others it requires little to no thought at all. Food is linked to our health and visual appearance and is always in the news.

If you are a bit like me, you may have been through different stages in your relationship with food: for example, changing your diet, strictly cutting out meals or doing the opposite and letting go because 'we only live once'. My relationship towards food has changed so many times, especially after reading about the new 'must have' superfood or about something you should no longer eat at all. In retrospect, I see that I was dependent on external sources rather than my own body when choosing what was best to put on my plate, and this approach never worked for long for me.

When I discovered mindfulness and started experimenting with it and incorporating it into different aspects of my life, I also started to eat mindfully. Over the first few months of the practice, my perspective towards food radically changed. It almost felt like I had never eaten before. I began to explore my inner dialogue with food and how I responded to the food I ate. Together with the body scan (refer to Chapter 4 for more on this), mindful eating became the most influential practice for me.

I would like to share more about my favourite mindful eating practices with you. Open your mind to this new way of experiencing food and enjoying the nourishment and energy that food naturally gives you.

Mindful Eating

Eating is an amazing way of practising mindfulness meditation, especially when you activate all your senses. You can try it alone, but my students and I find this practice more effective and enjoyable when experienced in pairs or groups (even a virtual group). My colleagues and I created a regular mindfulness lunch routine, and we all love it. You can organise different events with your friends or family to practise together (just imagine, a meal where there is no place for phones, only for the actual meal and fun). Fun is guaranteed! Read on to find out how you can start practising to become a Maestro of Mindful Eating.

Prepare three small pieces of a food that you like. You can choose grapes (my favourite), segments of tangerine, small cuts of apple, small cubes of chocolate or something savoury, like nuts. Find a nice quiet space and sit comfortably. Turn off your devices.

Take a few deep breaths to connect with your body. What are your feelings and thoughts? Are you hungry or do you feel quite full? Take the first piece of food you have prepared and simply place it on your palm. Imagine you are seeing it for the very first time in your life (fake it until you make it!). Observe the shape, colour, texture and weight on your palm. Take your time and be curious, as you never know when you may discover something new.

Then bring the food closer to your nose so you can smell it. The smell may cause you to want to eat it right away or it may awaken certain memories. Hold it to your ear, listen for any sound when touching the surface. You can also try to squeeze it a bit; do you hear anything?

Now place the food on your tongue: don't bite into it yet, but notice any instinctive urges to bite or swallow, and also note what is happening with your saliva. Move the food around your tongue and taste buds, and notice the different tastes and their intensity. Bite and notice the sensations on your teeth, the different textures and tastes. Don't rush, and take your time for every single bite. Observe what all your senses are experiencing as you bite into the food. Notice what your body urges you to do and how you can control your instincts when fully aware. After you have finished chewing, swallow the food and take a moment to follow the journey of the food through your body. Do you feel one piece of food fuller now? Now try the same thing with the remaining pieces.

Don't worry if you couldn't focus on all the aspects of mindful eating; the first experience can be quite overwhelming. You will build up your awareness with each practice and find what works best for you. Remember to have fun!

Mindful Food Shopping and Preparation

An important part of eating is what happens before we put food on our plate. When practising mindful eating, you become more aware of what types of food are nourishing for your body. You can try it the next time you go to the shop. Look at some food, hold it in your hands and think about whether eating it will make your body happy. Don't read the nutritional information, don't think about information you've learned from your friends or the media. Don't worry about the other people in the shop; they are busy with their own shopping. Ask yourself, how does this food make you feel when you smell it, look at it, hold it? What do your memories tell you about this food?

Try the same exercise at home as well. Try it when you feel hungry or have some cravings – before you unconsciously eat the first available thing, take a moment to ask your body how that food makes you feel. When cooking, use your senses to observe all the ingredients and be open to what your inner response is. Do you like the colours; is the smell appealing? Let your inner intelligence decide what is the best food for you.

It's also important to be mindful about where you choose to eat. Certainly, everyone has their own preferences, but you probably don't pay attention to them. Perhaps some of your meals are eaten at your desk or in front of the TV. Take a tour around your home and test a few places before finding the best one. Perhaps you love eating outside. Maybe you like to eat in the corner or facing the window, but you will never know unless you ask yourself.

Don't Forget to Get a Drink

As we all know, regular fluid intake is important, and drinking is another great mindfulness practice. Next time you're going to get something to drink, pay attention to how you feel before the first sip, while you are drinking, and after you have finished. Start regular thirst check-ups during the day and ask yourself how much you need to drink to stay hydrated.

I like to have a mindful moment when preparing my hot drinks. It starts when I take a cup, add a tea bag, fill up the kettle with water and press the button to heat it up. I consider all the changes from cold to boiling water by looking at and listening to it. Finally, I pour hot water over the tea bag. Depending on the time I have available, I sometimes continue with mindful drinking as well, paying attention to all the sensations. It is something you really can do anywhere, even at work. It is ideal for when you need to create time just for yourself, and it helps to improve focus because it is an activity that doesn't take too long (so you can concentrate during the whole process). Don't be limited to being mindful while making tea: you can be mindful preparing any drink, as well as any type of food.

Forbidden Fruit

Feeling regret and guilt after eating certain types of food, eating more than we should, raiding the fridge during the night and talking ourselves down for doing it again – let's be honest, we've all been there. We label our food as good or bad and we blame ourselves for eating the bad food. Give yourself a moment to think about what you are causing to yourself when you attach a negative message to the food you eat.

Try this simple exercise to discover your relationship with food:

- Write down everything you have eaten today.
- Add a tick next to all the meals you class as good, and a cross next to all you class as bad.
- Observe your feelings when reading the list.
- Consider how you would feel about sharing the list with others.

When practising mindful eating, you increase your ability to make conscious decisions about your food. Say, you are craving chocolate but the voice in your head is saying you shouldn't eat it. You try to think about something else, but chocolate appears in your mind again. Now, you have the option of pushing this voice down again, but, after some time, you act impulsively and you very quickly eat the whole chocolate bar, because you have deprived yourself for so long. A different option is to mindfully approach your chocolate craving and consciously treat yourself with a little piece of chocolate and slowly enjoy the rich cocoa taste.

Remember:

- Enjoy your meals and drinks with all your senses. Don't get too serious about your food and find time to experiment and play with it.
- Learn to understand the messages certain foods send to you. Listen to your body.
- Become an advocate of mindful eating practice, and encourage others to join you.

About Lucie Kysučanová

Lucie started practising mindfulness in the work environment, fell in love with it and became a mindfulness coach. She loves all areas of positive psychology and mindfulness and she enjoys sharing it with others. Her biggest inspirations are people, movement, nature and her cat Selma. She lives in London, UK.

www.lucie-kysucanova.com

11

Showing Ourselves Compassion

Stephanie Sackerman

If someone described you as compassionate, would you agree? Most people would say yes, yet how many of us truly embody the essence of compassion? It was only recently that I learned the true lesson of compassion: it starts with oneself.

It was just at the right moment in my life when I discovered the work of Kristin Neff, the leading researcher in the field of self-compassion. *Self-compassion* is when we respond to ourselves in the same way we'd respond to a friend or loved one when they've made a mistake or are having a difficult time. This is relevant for everyone because, as humans, we are bound to make mistakes. As a former perfectionist, I hate to admit it, but it's true: we are all flawed, and nobody is perfect.

This comes up a lot in the mindfulness coaching I do with parents. Anyone who is a parent, grandparent, guardian or caregiver knows the immense guilt that comes when you mess up. In my groups, we refer to it as 'Mom Guilt', but we've all felt it, or our own version of guilt. You know the feeling; when you criticise yourself and then ruminate over a mistake, robbing yourself of being in the moment. I often ask the parents I support if they would respond to their child in that same way when they're learning to walk and keep falling down. "Of course not!" is always the answer. Yet, we constantly do it to ourselves.

There are many reasons why we do this – unrealistic personal expectations, false societal expectations, childhood trauma, the quest for perfection, feelings of unworthiness; the list could go on – but one thing we can do to stop ourselves from responding critically is to begin practising self-compassion.

Bringing Mindfulness to Self-Compassion During Challenging Times

The first step is to become aware of our thoughts (hello, mindfulness practice!). One of my favourite things about mindfulness is that we are given the opportunity to respond to ourselves (and any outside situation or interaction) with kindness and non-judgement. Suddenly, we can have an uncomfortable thought or feeling, we can mess up and make mistakes, and we can be human. With mindfulness, we are given the chance to be compassionate to ourselves.

This is one of the greatest gifts mindfulness offers us when we find ourselves in uncertain times, with our nervous systems kicked into high gear. As a mindfulness teacher and a parent educator, I was completely devastated when on Day 20 of the coronavirus quarantine, I yelled at my toddler son. Afterwards, I replayed the moment over and over again in my mind, and I let my inner critic have its way with me. How could I, someone with such a strong mindfulness practice and positive parenting beliefs, have responded that way?

Then something wonderful happened: I remembered self-compassion. I paused for a moment, and I thought about all the emotions that I was feeling. I thought about the anxiety, fear, worry and stress that I – along with the rest of the world – was experiencing, and I gave myself grace. As disappointed as I was with myself, I knew how to return to the three elements of self-compassion (as outlined by Kristin Neff): mindfulness, common humanity and self-kindness.

Mindfulness. First, I acknowledged that this was a hard moment, made more difficult given the stressful circumstances, and I allowed myself to be aware of what I was thinking and feeling without judgement or shame. Our thoughts and emotions are meant to move through us without getting stuck; however, we often find ourselves trying to avoid a thought or deny a feeling and, as a result, we end up getting even more entangled with it. It's when we can acknowledge these thoughts and feelings, be with them, and respond to them with kindness that we can work through them. In this moment, I felt defeated, scared, frustrated and helpless, so I just let myself be present with these emotions.

Common humanity. Next, I remembered my humanness. As humans, we all experience emotions. What I'm experiencing has undoubtedly been felt before, and will be felt again by others. Life is not easy for anyone, and there is no need to ever feel alone. We are also connected in our universal needs. One of these is to feel safe and secure, but in uncertain times we can feel vulnerable and afraid, with our stress-response at code red. This doesn't mean that my reaction was right; it simply means that I am human, and I can allow myself to make mistakes.

Self-kindness. Finally, I responded to myself with kindness. Whether silent or aloud (given the moment and wherever we may be), we can simply speak lovingly to ourselves. My favourite phrases, which tend to resonate especially with parents, include: *May I be patient with myself, may I be kind to myself, may I forgive myself,* and *may I remember I'm doing the best I can.*

When I reflect on the interaction with my son through the lens of mindful self-compassion, I also invite myself to bring into awareness the emotions and thoughts in the moments leading up to and during it. Doing so helps us to be mindful of our own triggers. We all have triggers: things that elicit an emotional response with or without our conscious awareness. I've come to recognise that my trigger is feeling a lack of control. As humans, when we are triggered, we react in one of two ways: mindfully or instinctually. While I am usually able to respond in a mindful way, I responded in a more instinctive way in this example with my son. This recognition is not meant to excuse or justify my behaviour; it is simply to understand that in times of crisis, our survival instincts may surface, and we may find ourselves reacting in less helpful ways. Instead of responding critically, I can be compassionate with myself, take responsibility for my behaviour, understand why I responded that way, and move forward in a mindful way. For me, that means apologising to my son – explaining to him that sometimes Mommy gets upset (just like he does), and that I made a mistake (just like everyone does) – and then letting go.

It is in this letting go that we can show ourselves true compassion. This wasn't a lesson I always understood. As a new mother, I often criticised myself and felt like a complete failure. As a result, I was on an endless cycle of reacting in a way that I'd later be disappointed by, and then replaying the experience in my mind. Buddha called this the 'first and second dart'. The first dart, or arrow, is what actually happens. The second dart is what we continually throw at ourselves, reliving and analysing the situation – over and over again. In this way, we are often least compassionate with ourselves, which perpetuates the cycle of stress and suffering. When we instead shift towards a compassionate approach to ourselves, we can regulate our body's stress response towards a feeling of calm.

The amazing thing that happens is that as I practise giving compassion to myself, my compassion for others grows. What I practise on a daily basis strengthens, and so when I practise compassion for myself, it extends into my other relationships. But in order for us to be compassionate with others, the compassion must originate within ourselves.

A Self-Compassion Practice

One of the most well-known meditations is the loving-kindness meditation (or *metta* meditation). It starts by encouraging us to offer kindness to ourselves: *May I be peaceful. May I be happy. May I be safe. May I be loved.* The meditation then begins to pull a loved one into the mix: *May they be peaceful. May they be happy. May they be safe. May they be loved.* After that, the meditation begins to expand the focus: to an acquaintance, the local neighbourhood, the country or even the world.

The script varies, but the meditation tends to follow this order. This is important. Who is at the very beginning? It is you. If we want to send compassion, love and kindness out into the world – or simply give it to another person – we must first be able to give it to ourselves.

To do this, we must find what is comforting to us. For example, kind words, affirmations and loving self-talk fill me up. If your comfort is physical touch, then maybe you'd enjoy sending yourself compassion by giving yourself a squeeze, rubbing your arms gently to mimic a hug, or placing your hand over your heart. You might prefer to practise gratitude for yourself by surrounding yourself with a group of supportive and loving individuals who believe in you and help you to believe in yourself, or to shower yourself with love in another way. Whatever is comforting to you – and it may change! – the important thing is to be compassionate with yourself every single day, especially during uncertain times.

When you find yourself in a tough situation, follow these simple steps to help you be compassionate with yourself:

1. Pause and allow yourself to be present. Notice whatever it is that you are feeling and thinking without judging yourself or the emotion. Employing the first three steps of clinical psychologist Tara Brach's RAIN strategy is a beautiful way to do this:
    Recognise the thought or feeling.
    Allow whatever is happening to happen, without judgement or feeling the need to change it.
    Investigate whatever is happening with kind curiosity.
2. Honour yourself with supportive words: This is hard. This is a difficult moment. This is stressful.
3. Remind yourself that you are human, meaning that you're not perfect (nor is there a need for you to be). We all experience hardship, suffering and the consequences of our human flaws. At any given moment, there is probably at least one other person on the planet who is feeling the same way you are. Honour yourself with these comforting words: *Others have felt this way. No one is perfect. I am not alone.*

4. Give yourself the support and encouragement you need in the moment. Ask yourself, *What would feel good to me right now?* or *What do I need in this moment?* You may wish to employ the final step in the RAIN strategy here (Nurture with kindness), or to honour yourself with touch, connection or supportive words: *May I be patient with myself. May I be kind to myself. May I forgive myself. May I remember I'm doing the best I can. May I accept myself as I am.*

As you practise self-compassion, your body produces oxytocin and endorphins, reducing stress and increasing feelings of safety and happiness. With each practice of self-compassion, you are caring for yourself, reminding yourself of your value and worth, and cultivating a positive response to yourself – what could be better?

It is always helpful to practise self-compassion, especially in uncertain and stressful times. Honour yourself, your thoughts and your emotions by responding to yourself with the support and kindness that you would offer a friend or loved one.

I share a guided self-compassion meditation that you may find helpful: TeachMindfulnessOnline.com/book.

Remember:

- Self-compassion is showing ourselves the same kindness we would show a friend or loved one when they've made a mistake or are having a difficult time.
- Self-compassion allows us to respond to ourselves in a healthy way without giving us a 'pass' for our behaviour.
- It is when we give compassion to ourselves that we can best give compassion to others.

About Stephanie Sackerman

Stephanie is a certified educator, wellness coach and mindfulness teacher. She is passionate about supporting moms so they can stress less, love more, slow down to savour the moment, and show up as the moms they want to be. Stephanie's authentic approach focuses on mindfulness, kindfulness and compassion. She lives in New Jersey, USA.

www.LLBWC.com

12

Growing Gratitude

Laura Goren

A new client, Jenny, came to me for help. She said that she had everything she'd ever dreamed of: a loving husband, healthy kids, a successful career and a beautiful home. Despite all this, she felt unsatisfied. "I feel bleh about my life," Jenny said. "Why am I always seeing what I don't have? Why can't I just be happy with what's already here?"

Jenny's question struck me like an arrow into the heart. Firstly, because so many people experience similar struggles with dissatisfaction. Secondly, because I can relate. I, too, used to rest my happiness on the next big thing: "Once I get married, then I'll be happy... when we purchase a house, then I'll be happy... when I get that promotion, then I'll be happy." You, too, may relate to this belief that happiness is always just around the corner and overlook what you already have. *It is especially easy to overlook the good in life during difficult moments.* What we focus on grows, so when we focus on the negative, it is easy to get stuck there. Jenny was ready to get unstuck. She was able to do just that... by growing gratitude.

Understanding Dissatisfaction

Jenny's experience is common. Humans tend to look to the next big thing for happiness. Psychologists call this phenomenon the *hedonic treadmill*: if we can only achieve a little more, *then* we will be happy. However, according to this theory, human beings are exceptionally adaptable and whenever we get what we're seeking, it quickly becomes less valuable, so we return to our original baseline of happiness and the cycle repeats like a treadmill.

In addition, humans also have a tendency to focus on the negative. This is called the *negativity bias*. This tendency was an evolutionary advantage to our ancestors because by focusing on dangers, early humans could be prepared to face threats. That trait helped our human ancestors survive, and we inherited it. Today, we have the negativity bias, but we don't have the same threats. Instead of focusing on preparations for a tribal attack, modern humans might focus on scary news stories or, as in Jenny's case, on what's missing in life. The problem is that what we focus on grows stronger, and the more time we spend focusing on the negative, the more we get stuck in a loop of negative thoughts, feelings and behaviours. This loop could eventually manifest as general discontentment or even depression.

So, if humans spend a lot of time chasing the next big thing without experiencing greater happiness, what will satisfy us? If we have a natural tendency to focus on the negatives, what can people like Jenny do to appreciate all they have instead of always wishing for something else?

Mindfully Focusing on Gratitude

Fortunately, we can hop off this treadmill and relax the negativity bias. We can control what we focus on and we can *mindfully choose* to focus on *gratitude*! Gratitude is an appreciation of your world – both internal and external. It's a lens through which we can view any experience, and it can help orient us towards what we already have, instead of what we lack. Interestingly, you don't need to *feel* grateful to focus on gratitude. Just intentionally orienting yourself towards what you have in this moment will generate feelings of abundance.

Focusing on gratitude yields tremendous rewards. Grateful people are generally happy and healthy. In a review of research on gratitude, academics concluded that "gratitude has one of the strongest links to mental health and satisfaction with life of any personality trait – more so than even optimism, hope, or compassion… People who experience gratitude can cope more effectively with everyday stress, show increased resilience in the face of trauma-induced stress, recover more quickly from illness, and enjoy more robust physical health." Specifically, researchers showed that expressing gratitude improved wellbeing and health in college students and adults. Participants were asked to either count their blessings or their burdens. After a few weeks, the participants in the gratitude group had a more positive view of their life, experienced fewer symptoms of illness, and even spent significantly more time exercising. Based on this study, and many others, we've learned that focusing on gratitude can nurture positive states of mind and even encourage other healthy life choices. *Gratitude is self-care gold!*

It is worth mentioning that positive emotions like gratitude can make us resilient during particularly difficult times in life. Whether we are in the midst of a global pandemic or experiencing personal troubles, gratitude can be a vehicle for more positive states of mind. You may feel grateful that you still have your home, kind neighbours, even good weather! Biologically, gratitude can trigger releases of dopamine and oxytocin in the brain, hormones that help us feel optimistic, motivated and connected. When we can mindfully acknowledge that we are struggling, we can interrupt the negativity loop by inserting a gratitude practice. We have the power to create our own happiness loop!

Gratitude Practices

Viewing life through the lens of gratitude takes practice. Like riding a bike, the more you practice, the better you get at changing your perspective. You can get started right now with some of these fun practices. Commit to ones that resonate with you and see what you notice!

- **Good morning gratitude:** As soon as you wake up, spend two minutes writing down what you are grateful for. Try to linger on the way gratitude feels in your body as you write. Starting your day with a focus on what you are thankful for sets the tone for the rest of the day.
- **Squeaky clean gratitude:** Taking a morning shower? Let gratitude wash over you. Linger in appreciation of the warm water and soap. This turns an ordinary activity into a mindful moment of gratitude.

- **Gratitude pal:** Grab a small item like a pebble or cotton ball. Place it in your pocket and, every time you notice it throughout your day, use it as your cue to think of something to be grateful for.

- **Midday thanks:** Set an alarm to pause for gratitude. Think of someone who has enriched your life and thank them with a personal letter, email, phone call or text. Imagine their smile as they receive your message. Or, shine some light on yourself: what about yourself are you grateful for? Perhaps your strong body, forgiving heart or witty sense of humour?

- **Smile file:** Create a smile file on your phone or computer of images of things that you are grateful for. This file can also include inspirational songs, videos or poems that can spark a positive emotion like gratitude. Browse through it daily.

- **Gratitude reframe:** When you find yourself irritated by someone – a noisy co-worker or the pet who interrupts your mindful meditation – play with sending gratitude their way. Notice your irritation and then pause, relax your body, and think of how you are grateful for this being.

- **A grateful wait:** Turn moments of waiting (such as for water to boil or in a queue) into moments of gratitude. Think of what you could be grateful for in *this present moment*. You may feel grateful for your health, that you have some money for groceries, that you're wearing your favourite shoes. Your list might be longer than your wait. I share a three-minute guided grounding gratitude meditation that you might like to try: visit TeachMindfulnessOnline.com/book.

- **A-to-Zzzz:** Before falling asleep, think of one thing you are grateful for, for each letter of the alphabet. Warning: you may fall asleep by 'M'!
- **Gratitude journal:** Dedicate time before bed to write about what, on this day, you are thankful for. Fully describe your moments of gratitude and try to replay them in your mind. Be sure to linger in the feelings of warmth as you write.
- **Begin again:** Bookend your day with gratitude. Leave your night-time journal entry or gratitude list by your bed and read it when you wake up in the morning.

Gratitude meditation

In this practice, you set aside a longer period of time to explore the feeling of gratitude more deeply, including how it shows up in your physical body, breath, heart and mind.

To begin, find a comfortable position and close your eyes. Take a few deep, intentional breaths, and then allow your breath to fall into its natural rhythm. Feel the weight of your body seated or lying down. Then, bring to mind someone who you are truly grateful for and would like to thank. It could be a person or it could even be a pet. Picture this being in detail: the shape of their face, their eye colour. Now, say thank you in your mind: "Thank you, dear friend, for always being there for me" or "Thank you for believing in me." Imagine their face as you offer this appreciation.

Next, appreciate yourself. Tuning into the sensations of your breath, you can say, "Thank you, kind breath, for always being present for me. Thank you for your ability to soothe and relax me." And then tune into the sensations of your body and say,

"Thank you, kind body, for being here for me from the moment I was born. Thank you for doing your best to heal when you are hurt."

Next, perhaps with a hand on your heart, say, "Thank you, dear heart, for always being present and beating for me every second of my life." Then rest for a few minutes in the waves of breathing in gratitude and breathing out gratitude.

After you linger in these sensations of gratitude for as long as you like, begin to move your body again, and open your eyes.

Spend a moment now reflecting on that experience. Ask yourself how you felt at the end compared to the beginning.

I provide a guided audio track for this gratitude meditation that you may like to try: visit TeachMindfulnessOnline.com/book.

Gratitude Tips

Establishing a new way of looking at the world isn't easy. Here are some tips for growing gratitude:

- **Buddy system:** Find a friend who is interested in gratitude and explore together. This support can be helpful. If you are writing gratitude lists, you may consider taking a photo and sharing with your buddy.
- **Linger:** When you are practising, try to linger in the feeling of gratitude. Likewise, try to replay moments in your mind in detail. Spend some time exploring how that shows up in your physical body. This allows the brain's

neural networks to start recognising a new way of interpreting life.

- **Do it anyway:** Do the gratitude practices even if you don't feel grateful – sometimes you may feel irritated or despairing and gratitude seems out of reach. Practise anyway. Leaning towards gratitude can generate positive feelings of warmth and appreciation.

- **Use reminders:** Schedule time in your day to practise by setting an alarm on your phone, or sticking a note on the mirror to remind yourself to pause for gratitude.

Remember:

- Through the lens of gratitude, we intentionally appreciate what we have, rather than focusing on what we lack.

- By orienting ourselves towards gratitude, we cultivate positive states of mind that help us become more resilient, open, hopeful and optimistic.

- Everybody has personal preferences for gratitude practices, so it's important to find whichever practice resonates with you.

About Laura Goren

Laura Goren is a passionate and compassionate mindfulness practitioner. Laura's approach incorporates mindfulness practices through her company Zen Den Wellness. She is based in Livingston, New Jersey, USA.

www.zendenmind.com

13

The Power of Being Kind to Others

Sara Winiecki

Last week, when I was taking a walk down a neighbourhood sidewalk, a biker dude came up behind me and almost knocked me off my feet. Let's just say the neighbours saw me do an unflattering twirl that instantly transformed my look from boho chic to hot mess express.

After I got past the initial shock, I took a moment to stop and catch my breath. When I looked down, I saw colourful artwork made with chalk all along the road ahead. Many different parts of it were beautiful, but one portion really caught my attention. It was a simple sentence: "Smiles are contagious too."

From a distance, the world seems like a big, bad, scary place right now. If you watch the news and talk to the people around you, it is probably all about the coronavirus pandemic, or their anxiety about the future and fear of the unknown. While it is a time to take extra precautions, I'd also argue it's a time of great opportunity.

Kindness is coming out in the most unexpected ways. This is a time in history that will be remembered forever – something that we'll be asked about years from now: "What was it like?". It is my hope and my belief that we'll be able to tell stories not just of our pain and our struggles, but also of our resilience and our ability to come together with love and hope during unprecedented times.

Kindness is like a pop quiz for the soul. Life will ask you to be kind when you least expect it. You'll be challenged to step out of your comfort zone and extend the type of courage the world needs most. It's going beyond a superficial smile or sense of obligation. It's allowing your heart to open in such a way that it creates a shift within yourself and the people around you.

Think of it like this: you can learn about something in a classroom or in a book, but nothing can replace the understanding you get when you experience it for yourself. In other words, it's one thing to talk about what should be done to make the world a better place, and it's another thing to be an example of what you want to see in the world.

The Gift of Taking Action

One of the best pieces of advice I've ever received is this: "When you know someone is hurting, when you know someone is in need, act."

You may have heard people say things like, "I'm so sorry. I'm here to help if you need anything." While this is nice, I would encourage you to take it a step further. Don't wait to be asked: volunteer to help. You don't have to donate large amounts of money or commit to an excessive obligation. It could be as simple as calling someone on the phone just to say hi, bringing over a batch of homemade cookies, offering to watch someone's kids or sending someone flowers for no reason. These are simple but powerful actions.

When people are really struggling, when life has really got them down, they may be hesitant to ask for help. They may be afraid of being a burden, or worry that people will think less of them. That's why the gift of action is so powerful. You can show your love not because someone asked you to, but because it comes from the goodness of your own heart. The more you live with your heart, the richer you are.

In 2011, my mom was told she had a week to live. I remember sitting in that little white hospital room as the doctor explained that this was the end. As much as I wanted to burst into tears, I knew I had to keep it together – I was my mom's medical power of attorney. "Let's take her home, I know that's where she wants to be," I said.

My mom was so weak by that point that the hospital insisted that paramedics drive her home. So there I was, sitting in the back of an ambulance for the first time in my life, holding my mom's hand. As we approached her house, my mom looked up at me and said, "I'm not going to make it to Christmas this year, am I?" I didn't know what to say. December 25th was three weeks away.

A friend of the family heard about the situation and secretly got a group of people to come to the house to surprise my mom. They all arrived together, singing songs and carols as they decorated her bedroom. It was like Christmas had exploded all over the place, and it was awesome. The room was lit up with angels, garlands, lights, ornaments and, of course, a beautiful tree.

My mom passed away on December 9th, but Christmas came early for us that year because we were able to celebrate together.

All of us have the power through our words, experiences and actions to reach other souls: to inspire others and to touch their lives.

The Role of Perception in Being Kind

Spiritual teachers throughout the ages have taught us that our quality of life and state of mind largely comes from our perception: 90 per cent is how you react to things, while 10 per cent is what actually happens to you. It's like watching a movie with a friend. You can both watch the same movie at the same time and yet walk away with two totally different reactions and opinions.

Being aware of our perception is like having a secret code that unlocks ancient knowledge and new understanding. It allows us to begin cultivating mindfulness of our thoughts, our reactions and how we interact with other people.

Next time you get upset or frustrated, observe what it is that is causing you to become frustrated. Is your mind telling you that whatever is going on shouldn't be happening? Do you have all the facts, or are you making assumptions? What is it about this situation or this person that is triggering you and why? Try experimenting. Be aware of what your mind is doing. It is possible to handle every event by finding peace within yourself. And when you're able to find peace within yourself, you will be able to share that peace with others.

One day, when I first started travelling by myself, I was sitting at the airport terminal waiting for my plane. I'd been travelling all day and was drained by the crowds, the noise and the lack of good food. All I could do was stare at the clock on my phone, counting down the minutes to my departure.

You would think that the exhausted look on my face combined with my "I'm so over this" demeanour and generally gruff appearance would have turned people away, but one unexplainably energetic and happy woman threw her bag down right next to me and struck up a conversation.

In a thick Southern accent, she said, "Don't you worry now, everything's gonna be all right." She handed me a bottle of water and a silk eye pillow. "These are for you, honey," she said. "They'll make your travels a little easier. Sometimes the best thing we can do for everyone is to make sure we take good care of ourselves."

I think that what this kind woman taught me that day – when she looked beyond my demeanour and perceived how exhausted I was – can be applied to everyday life too. When we feel well rested, when our bellies are full, and when our needs have been met, we are more likely to show our best self to other people. In short, when we feel better, we do better.

In my experience, it's about making consistent conscious efforts to practise self-care while learning how to bring that same energy of love out into the world too. When you're kind to someone else and you share your happiness, you get more in return. In fact, many people say that they experience more happiness when they give something away than when they receive something for themselves.

If you've ever had the experience of having something kind done for you, you know how good it feels. If you've ever done something kind for someone else, you know it feels even better. It makes sense doesn't it? When we do good for others, it fuels all sorts of positive vibes.

The Benefits of Being Kind

Kindness is more than fluffy, gooey stuff that makes us feel good. Scientific evidence shows tangible benefits for both the giver and the receiver of any kind interaction.

Giving to others gives the human race back the one commodity that we're constantly in pursuit of: happiness. Here are some revealing statistics from US-based NGO Life Vest Inside and the Harvard *Social Capital Community Benchmark Survey*:

- People who give contributions of time or money are 42 per cent more likely to be happy than those who don't give.
- Spending on others feels better than spending on ourselves.
- Giving is linked to the release of oxytocin, a hormone that induces feelings of warmth, euphoria and connection to others.
- Children who learn and experience kindness tend to have stronger relationships with others because of their ability to empathise.

- Helping can enhance emotional resilience and can reduce the unhealthy sense of isolation. The health benefits and sense of wellbeing return for hours or even days whenever the helping act is remembered.
- Students who have *performed* acts of kindness with their peers, families and in the community had greater academic success than those who simply recorded *seeing* acts of kindness.

Believe it or not, one of the most common reasons people don't practise kindness is fear: fear of approaching a stranger, saying the wrong thing or simply not knowing what to do. An easy way to overcome this is with practice. Try taking a few risks to engage and support people in news ways. After all, it's usually when we step outside our comfort zone that the magic happens.

We are all trying to navigate our way through this world. Compassion and kindness arise from the awareness that we are more alike than we are different. In the same way you wish for happiness and health for your family, others do too. As you practise kindness and continue to extend kindness to yourself and the world around you, be reassured that you are not alone.

Compassionate and caring people all around the world are living examples of humanity at its best and the beauty that connects us all. For every one of us, there is something that you can do in your life, right now, to make a difference to the life of someone else. To extend yourself in kindness to anybody is an extension of kindness in the world. Incorporate more intentional acts of kindness in your life and see what happens. Perhaps it will make peacemakers of us all.

Remember:

- Taking kind action during times of difficulty can offer us an opportunity to change the course of our lives and the lives of the people around us.
- Engaging the power of perception helps us look for ways to move from bystander to changemaker through meaningful action and intentional kindness.
- Practising kindness is worth it: being kind has been shown to have many benefits that ripple out through the world.

About Sara Winiecki

Sara helps big-hearted professionals who are ready to find their purpose so they can create more income, more time, and more impact while living a life they love.

www.positivewellbeingonline.com

14

Micro-mindfulness Moments: Mindful Cleaning

Cheryl Green

Every day you have to deal with many aspects of your life: family, work, personal. You manage by juggling, prioritising, catching up and usually putting yourself last. But that's okay, you may think – that's just what your life is like at the moment, with lots of demands on you and your time.

Then you hit a really challenging time, perhaps in your personal or work life. It could be a demanding workload, illness or a change in your personal circumstances, such as a divorce or moving house. You feel physically and mentally exhausted and you simply don't know how you're going to cope.

You think you're a failure; people give you reassurance and advice, but nothing helps. You simply have too much to do and don't have time to fit in anything new to help the situation. You function on autopilot just to get things done.

This is an all too familiar tale. In my regular mindfulness groups, a number of people have caring responsibilities for elderly parents or look after grandchildren; others are working full time in stressful jobs with long hours. Others are working mothers with young children who describe their lives as "a hamster wheel". On top of that, you may have a critical voice that says things like, "You should be able to cope with that, you didn't do very well at that, why did you say that?" This is normal: it is sometimes difficult to be kind to ourselves.

In mindfulness terms you are in 'doing' mode and, to foster feelings of being able to cope, you need to get into more of a 'being' mode: simply being in the here and now and appreciating what you can.

In simple terms, 'doing mode' means getting involved with what is happening, be it analysing, overthinking or planning what to do next. 'Being mode' is being present and accepting of what is going on, in this moment. We have to spend periods of time in 'doing mode' to be able to function in life. But when there is so much to do and you don't get it all done, you get stressed – then you set goals and you don't always achieve them, so you become more stressed and are even harder on yourself. In 'doing mode', you're not connected with your senses in the present moment; instead, you're thinking about how things should be.

Finding Ways to Look After Yourself

Looking after yourself is really important, especially during challenging times. Nurturing a more compassionate approach to yourself, even for short periods of time, will encourage a better frame of mind to help you shift from 'doing' to 'being'.

Here are two simple things that you could try daily, even several times a day, which will help how you feel about yourself and your ability to cope.

- Take a few deep breaths and give yourself a hug; this releases oxytocin, the nurturing hormone, to make you feel better. Try and have a chuckle, releasing even more feel good hormones (like serotonin and endorphins), which reduce the stress hormones and make you feel good.
- Consider what you would say to a friend who shares with you what their critical voice says to them, and how they feel overwhelmed and stressed. Now be that friend, but to yourself. Speak encouragingly to yourself and be your own best friend. Show compassion to yourself.

Part of mindfulness is to experience more 'being' moments in your daily life. 'Being mode' is about being in touch with the present moment, connecting with your senses of sound, smell, sight, taste and touch. You can try to accept things as they are and also cultivate gratitude (refer to Chapter 12).

You might understandably think, "How am I going to fit this into my overstretched life, when I feel I have barely got time to breathe?" To be mindful, you don't have to have a set amount of time that you must practise for. You can bring more 'being' and mindful moments into your life by doing some everyday tasks in a mindful way. You can have micro-mindfulness moments throughout your day; for example, when cleaning.

Mindful Cleaning

Cleaning is something that we all do, be it washing ourselves, our clothes, our car, our home... it is a core component of our lives. During the challenging time of the coronavirus pandemic, cleaning seems to have taken centre stage because we want to keep ourselves and our loved ones safe.

In times of illness or the threat of illness, or living with someone who is vulnerable, we tend to clean even more. If, like many, you see cleaning the home as an evil necessity, it can add more pressure to an already busy life.

Bringing mindfulness into your daily cleaning practice gives you the benefits of mindfulness, while also improving your everyday wellbeing – without you having to add extra activities or tasks into your busy life.

Here are some examples of how you can bring some daily micro-mindfulness moments into your life, while doing everyday tasks.

Vacuum cleaning

Decide which area you want to clean.

Observe how dirty the area is, and whether there are objects that you could move so that you can focus on just vacuuming without interrupting the flow of movement.

Take a few deep breaths, switch on the vacuum cleaner, and notice the sounds it makes.

Rhythmically move the vacuum cleaner across the floor.

Listen to the sounds, and look at any patterns that the hoover make on the floor as you move it. Do the sounds change? You might want to develop a rhythm of movement and notice how that makes you feel.

When you have finished, spend a few minutes looking at the clean floor.

Express gratitude that you have a vacuum cleaner that helps make the work easier.

Wiping work surfaces

Take a few deep breaths.

Clear the surface that you are going to wipe.

If you're using a spray cleaner, shake the bottle and look at the bubbles that you've created.

Spray the surface, notice the fragrance of the cleaner, and look at the patterns that form on the work surface.

Wipe the surface with a clean cloth. You may wish to create a pattern of movements as you wipe the surface clean: across, up and down.

Watch the surface dry.

Express gratitude that you can easily clean your work surfaces for preparing food.

Personal Hygiene

Here are some suggestions for creating some daily micro-mindfulness activities. Depending on how long you wish to spend on mindful tasks, you might only include some of the suggested activities – or you can add your own.

Cleaning your teeth

Here's an opportunity for a few minutes of mindfulness while brushing your teeth at the start and end of your day.

Take a couple of deep breaths.

Look at your toothbrush: the colour, the shape, the bristles. Turn it over to look at the back and the sides.

Pick up the toothpaste and look at the tube. What does it feel like to touch? Squeeze the paste on the brush and notice what it looks and smells like.

Begin brushing your teeth, and notice what the brush feels like in your mouth. *Taste the toothpaste.*

Loosen your grip on the toothbrush. Feel the bristles moving over your teeth and gums.

Do the bristles feel the same in all parts of your mouth? Don't worry if you don't notice any difference, that's just how it is for you at this moment.

After you rinse, take a few deep breaths. Notice your clean teeth.

Express gratitude for your teeth, and all that they enable you to do: chew, smile, speak.

Taking a mindful shower

Taking a shower is a great way to engage all of your senses in a mindful way.

Take a few deep breaths.

Listen to the sound of the water. What patterns and sounds does it make as it sprays onto the floor of the tray or bath?

Smell your soap, body wash and shampoo.

Now turn your attention to your body. Feel the temperature of the water on your skin. What does it feel like when you wash your body? Focus on your movements and the sensations you experience. Try washing yourself in a different way than you normally would.

Just like you would in regular meditation, take a moment to breathe in and out. Close your eyes and let the water gently run over you.

Express gratitude as you shower, feeling thankful for the hot water, the soap and the pleasure of being clean. Acknowledge all that your body does for you.

Mindfully washing your hands

Take a couple of deep breaths.

Turn on the tap, and notice how the water feels on your hands.

Put soap on your hands, rub your hands together and notice how the soap lathers – how your hands feel as the soap cleans them. What do you notice?

Rinse your hands.

Gently dry your hands, noticing how the towel feels on your skin.

Give gratitude for having soap and water to be able to wash your hands.

I share a guided audio version of this mindful activity that you may like to follow: visit TeachMindfulnessOnline.com/book.

Remember:

- You are not alone in your thoughts and feelings of being overwhelmed; throughout the world, there are people who feel exactly like you.
- Mindfulness is about kindness and compassion to yourself.
- Mindfulness is not just meditation; you can be present by doing everyday tasks such as cleaning, which can help to improve your sense of self-acceptance.

About Cheryl Green

Cheryl is a certified mindfulness and laughter therapy teacher interested in self-compassion and applying mindfulness in everyday life. She loves penguins! She is based in Bedford, UK.

15

Mindfulness for Finding Joy

Jennifer Gilroy

You only need to search the word 'joy' in a dictionary to find a huge list of beautiful words, such as 'glee', 'elation', 'rapture'. Joy is not necessarily a simple, singular feeling, but an array of mental states, feelings and bodily sensations. Joy is appreciation, contentment, gratitude. It is the feeling of vitality, of being alive, of being glad. It is the very essence of tenderness; it is openness of heart. Joy is also expressed within our laughter.

We all have the potential, and capacity, to live life more happily again. And we can do it simply, by practising mindfulness. So, my friend, I will do my best to show you how.

When we practise mindfulness – when we sit down to meditate, or walk mindfully, or eat mindfully – we are both training and cultivating ourselves simultaneously. We develop our attention as we move through the practice. We become aware, we are aware, and in turn we develop intrinsic human qualities that enable us to put our trust into life, to take a step back, and to feel contentment. In the same way, joy can be trained and cultivated. We need joy within our lives: it should be there in equal measure to all the other emotions that we experience. We can also investigate why we lack joy.

Enabling the Conditions Where Joy Exists and Grows

Within our mindfulness journey, we come to realise that the joy and fulfilment we seek comes from being in the present moment. But, my friend, we live in such a hectic world, and somehow we don't, or can't, allow ourselves to be fulfilled by normal everyday things. Even when it comes to such a nice thing as relaxing! We spend around 50 per cent of our time thinking about the past or future, and we spend it there for plenty of reasons. We might regret something that has happened, or we might worry about something that is yet to happen. We wonder about the past and the future. We fear both. However, the act of being in the past or the future is also linked to attachment.

Attachments (also referred to as cravings) are the things, ideas and thoughts that we fixate upon. The notion that we should be rich. The perfect holiday that will surely happen because we have planned it so well. We fixate, and we attach. This is where we ought to be. This is how things should go. These attachments are formed by our thoughts, and historical mindfulness teachings refer to these as 'objects of the mind'.

So, attachments are the things that we fixate on, and if we fixate then we cannot be present. If we are not present, then we cannot find joy.

One of the main purposes of mindfulness is to reduce our suffering. Attachment, especially to something unachievable, or to something that we don't have, causes such suffering. If we want to enable the conditions where joy can exist and grow, then we can investigate this form of suffering. Spend a while quietly contemplating what you are attached to. You may be surprised at what comes up for you. Take your time, meditate on things. Might you gather insight and decide that loosening your grip on these attachments could be a powerful thing? Could it be that you decide that allowing things to take their natural course will reduce your suffering even more? Could you, over time, become more open to the availability of joy, perhaps even the idea of residing in a joyful place?

We are all at different stages within our mindfulness journeys. So, my friend, I want to give you some practical practices that you can use, even if you are new to mindfulness.

The Joy of Eight Breaths meditation

This is a beautiful meditation that can help to remind us that life is there to be enjoyed. You can practise by spending some time focusing on each area, or by reciting each word on each breath. I like to spend some time focusing on each area, before moving on to a few rounds of reciting.

With each area, you can repeat the word to yourself. You may like to use an app such as Insight timer (which includes guided meditations and an adjustable personal timer) to set your rounds so that you can keep track.

Take some time to settle into a comfortable position. Ground yourself, lower your gaze or close your eyes, and relax. You may like to take a few deep, mindful breaths and relax your shoulders further as you breathe out.

1. **Breath.** Bring your awareness to your breathing. Allow yourself to breathe naturally; no control is required. Simply follow your in-breath and your out-breath.
2. **Body.** Bring your awareness to everything that you notice within your body. Each and every sensation. Notice the good feelings, and the not-so-good. Keep in mind any discomfort you feel.
3. **Release.** Imagine that you can release all the tension and discomfort within your body on your out-breath.
4. **Cravings.** Notice whether you are happy to accept things as they are. Notice any tendency to want things to be different within your life.
5. **Love.** Here, lend some love and compassion towards yourself. Wish yourself ease of being.
6. **Letting Go.** Become aware that all of the right conditions to bring you happiness and joy are already here. We were born with nothing; what do we really need? For every reason to suffer there is a reason to be joyful, and what matters is where we choose to focus our attention.
7. **Alive.** Become aware that you are alive. Recognise how precious your life is. Feel alive.
8. **Beauty.** Consider the beauty that is all around you, and within you.

You may find that by now your breath has slowed as your body has relaxed and your mind has become focused. If you wish, you can recite the words as you breathe, in the same order, one word for each in- and out-breath, finishing the meditation when you are ready.

Appreciative Joy

This is a practical exercise that can help bring joy into your life through appreciation. Like writing a gratitude journal, the act of being appreciative naturally encourages us to become happier as people.

Spend some time, perhaps once a day, being truly appreciative. Do everything and experience everything with an open heart. Become aware of the generosity that is given and received. Feel into an appreciative world. Let appreciation occur in the smallest of happenings – how your partner chose to give you the largest portion of dessert; the birds singing; hearing your child breathe as they fall asleep.

Beginner's Mind

American Professor Jon Kabat-Zinn recognised a number of 'attitudinal foundations' of mindfulness. These foundations are both elements of, and fruits of, mindfulness practice. As you move forward on your mindfulness journey, you might wish to research these online. This exercise takes into account one of these foundations: the Beginner's Mind, an attitude of seeing things afresh.

Bring your awareness to an everyday thing that you enjoy, perhaps preparing and drinking tea. See if you can intentionally become completely aware as you carry out this task, but with an air of sensitivity, of receptiveness to the pleasure and enjoyment of this simple thing, as if it is completely new to you. Notice, if you can, how wholeheartedly experiencing the moment can enhance feelings of joy.

Peace and Freedom meditation

I would like to share with you a guided Peace and Freedom meditation, one that you can listen to on those days when you might like to enjoy a beautiful, calm, open and peaceful space (visit TeachMindfulnessOnline.com/book).

These are my tips to you, as I write this during the coronavirus pandemic in 2020. I encourage you to feel comfort during these times. Our life paths have always been uncertain – is there anything that is different now? I wish you well, and I wish you joy.

Remember:

- Joy is best found when we enable the conditions where it can exist and grow.
- Understand suffering: how it relates to the absence of joy, and how we can curiously investigate it.
- Use the practices in this chapter for exploring, encouraging and cultivating joy.

About Jennifer Gilroy

Jen is a mindfulness teacher based in Surrey, England. You can contact her by visiting her Facebook page (@ZenJenmindfulliving), and you can also find her on Instagram.

16

Connecting with Nature

Clare Snowdon

At times in my life when I have faced stress or a difficult challenge, I have found peace, and often a solution, by 'taking the problem for a walk' – either by sitting on a hillside, watching the view and feeling the wind on my face, or simply by putting one foot in front of the other until my mind becomes quiet. The sight of people in parks during the coronavirus crisis suggests that I am not alone in finding comfort in nature. In fact, it seems that connecting with nature is an essential part of our wellbeing.

What Is Nature Connection?

Much of our experience of nature involves activities in green spaces – often walking, playing, or having a picnic. It might involve feeding the ducks or bird spotting. These activities involve *contact* with nature but not necessarily *connection*.

There are certainly benefits associated with contact with nature. Plants emit immune system-boosting chemicals called *phytoncides* which are used in some aromatherapy oils. Researchers at the University of Bristol have even discovered a microbe in the soil that may help to reduce symptoms of depression! So, simply investing time in nature can have a positive effect on our mental and physical wellbeing.

Nature connection or *natural mindfulness* is far more about the 'felt' experience of nature than it is about our knowledge of or simple exposure to the natural environment. In short, connecting with nature deepens and reinforces the experience of being in nature. It's a bit like a visit to a museum. When we walk round a museum, reading the facts and looking at the exhibits, it can certainly be interesting or even amusing. However, when we start to empathise with historical figures (maybe putting ourselves in the shoes of someone living in the Middle Ages, or feeling for ourselves what it might have been like for an inventor to see the outcome of their work), the experience is much richer. We are perhaps able to engage much more of ourselves and our human experience.

Where Does Mindfulness Come into It?

Arguably, without mindfulness, any kind of connection is impossible. Imagine having a conversation with someone, but your mind is somewhere else – you are not really listening. We have all done this at some point in our lives. When we are not listening, we are not connected with the person who is talking to us, and it is very much the same with nature connection. In order to connect, we need to bring awareness. Luckily, we can be mindful of nature very easily, often without even intending to be.

Suppose that a deer suddenly runs across your path when you're out on a walk. I would not imagine, at that moment, that you'd be thinking of your to-do list. Instead, the deer has your full attention and has drawn some gentle curiosity from you. You may be aware of feeling more alert, possibly even aware of the sound of your breath, or the feeling of your pulse as you try to remain still and quiet. This is a moment of connection and mindfulness.

Most of the time with nature connection, we don't experience such a strong and attention-grabbing moment as this, so it is necessary to adopt a mindful approach, which may take a little practice.

Why Practise Mindful Nature Connection?

Investing time in nature offers many physical and mental health benefits. Even listening to recordings of birdsong or seeing pictures of nature have been shown to have a positive effect. The benefits include lowered blood pressure; enhanced immune system function, recovery from illness and reduction of pain; and the relief and possible prevention of the symptoms of depression and anxiety (scientific research suggests that experiences in nature reduce rumination, which is a key factor in depression and anxiety). However, what brings me and many others back to nature time and again is far harder to measure. There is a sense of belonging, of not being alone, even when we are the only people around for miles. A feeling of 'coming home' is commonly reported, as well as a sense of joy and deep relaxation.

I first truly noticed the benefits of connecting with nature when I was housebound for a period of time. I started to struggle with low mood. I decided to try walking a 30-minute loop from my home, taking in a local park with a river and some small wooded areas. The combination of the birdsong in the trees and the sunlight dancing on the surface of the water had an almost immediate effect. I caught myself smiling and noticed a heart-warming sense of joy starting to flood my body.

Some Suggested Practices

There is no 'right' way to practise mindful nature connection, as long as you are kind and respectful of all nature (including yourself and other people), so experiment and have fun! You are aiming for an awareness of what is 'here' – inside and outside of you. It's simple, but not always easy!

I always start by stopping. Even if the intention is to walk in nature, I start by standing still. I take a few deep breaths and notice my breathing as a process of nature and also an exchange. Breathing is a life process; a sequence of many, many activities, all working together to transport the things you need into your body and some of the things you do not need back out again. The oxygen you breathe comes largely from plants, which also use the carbon dioxide we breathe out. So, with every breath, we are both a living embodiment of nature and part of an interconnectedness with other organisms. Just by being and breathing, you are an essential part of the cycle of life on Earth.

You can choose to stay with the experience of breathing and reflect on it. It is a mindful practice in itself – just breathing with nature. (Resting against a tree and breathing is a lovely way to connect with nature, and I have provided some audio guidance to do just that at TeachMindfulnessOnline.com/book.)It is also a nice way to bring yourself to the present moment before moving to the next part of the practice.

I might next notice the earth beneath my feet. Your body is supported and held, in every moment, by a whole planet. It is good to take some time to notice the ground beneath you, and the feeling of being supported and held. You could even sit or lie down on the ground to feel what that is like.

The possibilities from here are almost endless. You could choose to sit or lie in your chosen place. This is known as a *sit-spot* practice. I have a sit-spot in my garden that I return to most days. Alternatively, you could start walking, slowly and mindfully, taking things in as you go, and pausing when you are drawn to do so. You may not get very far, but that is not the purpose of the walk.

Whether you are sitting or walking, continue to follow your breathing as you notice the ground beneath you. You can also open up your senses further. Listen to the sounds around you – allow all the sounds to 'land' on you, including the man-made ones, remembering that people are part of nature too. You may notice yourself judging or thinking about the sounds – some sounds you might find pleasant, while you might find others unpleasant and wish they weren't there. Invite some curiosity towards those feelings, and see if you can explore what those sounds are like without judgement. Does your experience of them change? What do you notice most strongly, and are you able to 'tune through' the sounds, a bit like listening to the radio, where some things may move into the background, while others come to the foreground.

It is lovely to notice how the sounds fit together like a piece of music, as well as to include any sounds you make yourself (such as your breath, or the sounds of any movement). When I walk, I like to map out the 'soundscape' of my journey. Try noticing how each part of your journey sounds or feels to you. If you have started from a built-up area or road, this may feel different to a later part of your walk, but it might also feel quite different when you walk back towards your starting point.

You can do the soundscape activity with other senses too (maybe air temperature or scents) and also by connecting with a general gut feeling. I love to pause and ask myself, "How does this place feel to me?" Sometimes it will feel peaceful or cool, or dark or busy. Noticing your feelings and what emotion or body sense is connected with your present moment experience is an important part of nature connection. You could even make a map at the end of your walk, with 'landmarks' based on your experience rather than physical objects – it could be something like the smell of a moss-covered log; a still, peaceful spot; or where you climbed a mound like a child to be the king or queen of the castle! The map will be different every time, even if you follow the same route on your walk.

Finding a Natural Mindfulness Guide

There are many natural mindfulness guides who can guide you on an experience near to where you live (or online, for example at https://natureconnection.world/). This allows you to share your experience with others and get different perspectives, which is a very powerful part of any mindfulness practice. Even as a guide myself, I benefit greatly from joining other guides and allowing myself to experience nature through their connection with it.

Other activities you can try include:

- Listening to birdsong recordings – even five minutes a day has been shown to have a beneficial effect
- Paying close attention to a natural object such as a stone, pot plant, pine cone or feather (my three-minute audio practice at TeachMindfulnessOnline.com/book may be a helpful guide)
- Growing something – maybe some wildflower seeds or herbs in a window box
- Watching the birds or clouds, or looking at the stars
- Noticing the weather or changes in the seasons
- Connecting with a pet
- Going camping – even in your own garden – as a kind of mini retreat

Remember:

- We are nature – we are not separate from it!
- Nature connection has many physical and mental wellbeing benefits and is a very accessible path to mindfulness.
- There is no 'doing it right'. Even distracted time in nature has benefits, and it can be helpful to practise nature connection when your mind is busy or stressed. Consider this Zen saying: "You should sit in nature for 20 minutes a day… Unless you are busy, then you should sit for an hour."

About Clare Snowdon

Clare trained to teach mindfulness in 2016, and trained as a natural mindfulness guide in 2019. She's based in London, UK.

http://dragonmindfulness.co.uk/

17

Mindful Movement in Nature

Lauretta Mazza

'Note from Shamash: To conclude this part of the book on practising self-care, compassion and kindness, and to follow Clare Snowdon's insights on connecting mindfully with nature, I hope you enjoy this poem from Lauretta Mazza, which captures the spirit and beauty of being in nature. Listen to Lauretta's two guided movement meditations at TeachMindfulnessOnline.com/book.

Brand New Day

It's a brand new day; let's take a walk outside, a mindful walk.
Stretching, yawning in the fresh air of the morning, what a blessing!
Wherever you are in the world, if it's summer, winter, full sunlight or still a little bit dark, let's start with a few steps.

Barefoot or wearing shoes, we start slowly, one step at a time, feeling the connection with the soil.
It's a very slow walk, trusting the support from our feet, like baby steps, looking for balance.
And what if our feet were like hands caressing the earth?
How could it be easier?
Step by step, in slow motion, we start to feel a little rhythm rising up.
It's our own rhythm, connected to the breath, synchronising steps and breath in a natural way, shifting the weight from side to side in an easy flow.

We can then shift our connection to the outside, to the gentle sound of our steps on the ground, to the freshness of the air on our skin and to the beauty that surround us.
With soft and round eyes that caress everything we see, we receive the light, the colours, the form of the different trees, bushes, flowers, stones, wild berries.
We can meet here a perfect match between the internal sensations of the breath, and the external sensations of the light and colours.
We choose the first colour we see and breathe, nurturing the entire body with that colour, exhaling what we don't need anymore – carbon dioxide, thoughts.

We can come to a place that we like, where it's nice to stand, receiving all the sounds around us: the birds, the wind, maybe water flowing somewhere.
Feeling the roots under our feet and the connection to the sky.
Here, feet apart at the same width as our pelvis, we start to turn, letting the arms be free to swing from side to side, centring our body and our emotions.
Standing or lying on the grass, a nice body scan can start from your feet and continue to your legs, pelvis, torso, hands, arms,

shoulders, neck and head, feeling the warmth and light of the sun enter into our bones, deep inside.

We can then land our attention on our breath again, inhaling the beauty that surrounds us and exhaling our inner peace.
And if we see water, a lake or a puddle, we can perceive the reflections of the light, stay and contemplate the water as a reflection of our mind.
How do you feel?
Take a big breath, smell the moment and have a good day!

About Lauretta Mazza

Lauretta is a Trager practitioner, and teaches the Franklin Method, Nia: Moving to Heal and mindfulness. Lauretta runs courses for individuals, companies, communities and small groups in both Italian and English. She lives in Tuscany, Italy.

www.in-movimento.org

www.trager.it

PART 3
CONNECTING MINDFULLY WITH OTHERS

18

Mindful Communication in Challenging Times

Calvin Niles

Think about someone in your life that you love dearly. What was the last thing you said to them, and the last thing they said to you? Was your communication built on a strong foundation of understanding? Was it kind? Respectful? Compassionate?

Mindful communication can be described as communicating in a way that encompasses the overarching principles of mindfulness. Encompassing Jon Kabat-Zinn's definition of mindfulness, these principles include "paying attention, on purpose, in the present moment and non-judgementally". Since paying attention requires intention, you can say that mindful communication brings greater awareness to the attitudes we bring to our communication, how deeply we listen, and how we express our thoughts and feelings.

Communicating during a Crisis

As you read these words, people all over the world will be experiencing difficulty, a big societal challenge or even a deep crisis. Billions of people have been asked to stay at home during the unprecedented coronavirus pandemic sweeping the world: a crisis of such magnitude that the economic and social effects may be felt for generations. Emotions will already be heightened by worries about the future, with the physical lockdown only amplifying people's fears. You may be experiencing some of these things yourself.

Our relationships and the way we communicate with each other can suffer greatly in times of crisis. During challenging times, the people around us – our partners, our children, the ones we care for most – are the ones who bear the brunt of our stresses when we aren't able to communicate effectively. Communication is the lynchpin upon which a healthy society rotates, and it is the fundamental basis of our connection with each other. Building better ways to communicate matters, but doing so mindfully is especially important in difficult times.

Cultivating Presence

One of the benefits of practising mindfulness is presence. You can think of presence as 'being here now, and staying here now'. The steadiness of your mindfulness, or the extent to which you can sustain your awareness, determines how present you are when you communicate. It may help to think of presence as the nurturing soil to help grow the seeds of mindful communication. To create that nurturing environment, meditation – the central practice of mindfulness – is key.

The body is a vital part of our awareness of the present moment, which is why re-connecting with the body and our sensory awareness is the basis of mindfulness meditation. It is especially important to keep in touch with what is going on within us as our emotions flow through the body. As you develop mindfulness through practices such as the body scan, you train yourself to deepen your presence in each moment. I share a guided body scan meditation that you can use as part of your meditation practice. I also provide a short meditation that you can use throughout your day to anchor you to the present moment. Visit TeachMindfulnessOnline.com/book.

The Seeds of Mindful Communication

"Speak briefly, speak warmly, and fill every sentence with kindness, clarity, and optimism." Mark Waldman

Communication is always taking place. However, when we are mindless with our communication, our messages can be diluted and misconstrued at best, or untimely and malevolent at worst – all of which can be amplified by a crisis. Seeding your communication with mindfulness allows you to bring helpful attitudes, listen deeply and express yourself in a way that is timely and constructive.

Attitude! Set your intention, give your attention

Have you ever reflected on the attitude that you brought to a conversation with someone? Or considered the power of bringing a chosen attitude to your communication in advance? When we find ourselves in difficulty, our heightened emotions can cause our autopilot mode to take charge of the way we communicate. However, by bringing certain mindful attitudes to bear, we make an active and intentional choice about the way we speak and listen.

Consider how these nine mindful attitudes might play a significant role in helping you to communicate more mindfully:

- **Beginner's mind.** Viewing things with a sense of curiosity can help to open the doorway to the perspective of the other person and, by extension, open up new levels of understanding.

- **Patience.** Feeling at ease about letting things happen in their own time allows the other person the space to experience their thoughts and feelings – without being pressured by you to wrap up or shut up!

- **Trust.** Trusting in your own experience, in yourself and your feelings, helps you to respect the other person's experience as being equally valid.

- **Non-striving.** Being at ease in the present moment without doing or trying to achieve a particular goal allows for freedom of communication between yourself and others, with no predefined outcome.

- **Non-judging.** Being the witness to your moment-by-moment experiences opens new pathways of listening and expressing yourself that are not coloured by your desire to label things as 'good' or 'bad'.

- **Acceptance.** Seeing things for what they are, without wishing they were different, creates the space and openness for communication to take place. It acts as a lubricant for positive changes to occur.

- **Gratitude.** Focusing your attention on all the good things in your life leads to positive feelings that translate to high regard for the people you're communicating with.
- **Generosity.** Honouring your partner with your presence and your full, unconditional attention is a great gift.
- **Letting go.** Releasing your mental or emotional grip on anything, whether a person or an experience, grants a freedom to your communication so that it flows effortlessly through the stream of mindfulness.

To explore how these attitudes, contribute to mindful communication, try reflecting on the last meaningful conversation you had with a loved one. How effective were you at applying these attitudes?

Deep listening

One of the greatest respects you can pay someone is to give them your full attention. With an attitude of generosity, you give the gift of deep listening. While listening requires that you focus your attention on what the other person is saying, deep listening adds the mindful dimension of presence, where you can listen patiently, trustingly and without judgement to both the speaker and yourself. It extends to what is not being said as well as what is being felt. With presence, being able to listen to your partner as well as to what is going on within you is of equal value.

When you listen deeply and create the space for expression (the third seed of mindful communication, which is discussed in the next section), you have the power to deflate much of the angst that a crisis generates. However, developing your mindfulness practice and cultivating your presence doesn't make you suddenly superhuman! We all become distracted at times, especially during difficult times, so re-establishing your connection with the present moment whenever you become distracted will help you to continue listening deeply. But sitting in the lotus position with your eyes closed and meditating is probably not the best thing to do mid-conversation! Fortunately, you can return your focus to the present moment in other ways.

A 'now anchor' can be helpful to bring you back to present-moment awareness. The breath is often used as an anchor because it's with you all the time. You may also choose to use an external anchor, such as a simple object (perhaps a stone, a vase or an ornament, or even part of the other person's body). It will help you bring your attention back to the present moment. Whenever your mind strays, say to yourself, "wandering!" and refocus on your chosen now anchor.

Don't be discouraged by the number of times you need to re-establish presence when you're listening. You may have to anchor yourself many times during a mindful conversation, which is perfectly okay. It is akin to doing reps in the gym: the more you do, the stronger you get!

To explore how listening deeply can enhance mindful communication, try setting your intention to listen intently during your next conversation with someone. Choose a 'now anchor' to help you return to present-moment awareness when you need to. It may help to journal on how deeply you feel you listened, and if any other challenges arose for you during the conversation.

Compassionate expression

French composer Claude Debussy once said that "music is the silence between the notes." Music can be a beautifully transformative form of expression and is a source of inspiration for many people enduring challenging times. Yet without the silence between the notes, music would simply be a cacophony of noise.

Compassionate expression can be just as transformative. If we are able to punctuate our own communication with silence, the silence can become harmonious with presence because it deters mindlessness when we communicate. Silence gives us the space to be compassionate when we speak. Bringing the attitudes of non-judgement and acceptance to our communication smooths the path we need to walk to embrace our feelings and sit in the warm glow of self-compassion (read Chapter 11 for more about self-compassion). This glow brightens when we speak, and its rays shine onto the other person and help open them up to full bloom.

Imagine it is your turn to speak. Ask yourself: Is what I am about to say timely? Am I in the right place to express what I want to say? Who is around me? Is the other person receptive at this moment? *Timeliness* means considering the moment you are in, along with what you want express and its ramifications. It is about giving yourself the best opportunity to be understood. Presence helps to bring insight to the timeliness of your communication because it is just as much an intuitive judgement as it is a rational one. You can assess constructive communication by asking yourself: How does what I want to say help overall? Does it build the person up or tear them down? Will it illuminate a new perspective for me and them? Will it encourage them to be open?

Compassionate expression is kind. Compassionate communication is gentle. A calm voice soothes. Speaking slower and at a lower volume lends itself to softness. When we express ourselves compassionately, we dissolve the barriers that exist between us and we reunite with our common desire to be loved, heard and understood.

To explore the impact of compassionate expression on mindful communication, you may like to reflect on another conversation you have had recently. Did you express yourself compassionately? Journal on where you feel you expressed yourself compassionately and where you feel you didn't. Note down the feelings you experience.

Every day provides us with new opportunities to communicate more mindfully. As you learn to apply these principles to your communication, your relationships will take a huge leap in a positive direction. Combined with your meditation practice, you can use the LEAP acronym to help you integrate the seeds of mindful communication at any time:

Listen deeply

Express yourself compassionately

Attitude! Bring mindful attitudes to bear

Presence is key

Remember:

- During times of crisis, our communication can become mindless and the people around us may suffer. Mindful communication can help us during challenging times.

- When mindfulness is sustained, we have presence. Meditation is key to establishing presence, which allows us to cultivate the conditions for healthy communication.
- Setting an intention to bring a mindful attitude to your communication, to listen deeply, and to express yourself compassionately, are the three essential seeds for nurturing mindful communication with everyone.

About Calvin Niles

Calvin uses mindfulness in his coaching to empower others to discover their key message, share their story and communicate with impact. He lives in London, UK.

www.calvinniles.com

19

Connecting with Others Online

Melissa Acuna-Dengo

"We are biologically, cognitively, physically, and spiritually wired to love, to be loved, and to belong." Brené Brown

We have all felt it. That powerful energy exchange that happens between people who are truly present with one another. Who have given their entire attention to this other person and allowed themselves to be seen. This, my friends, is what we call connection.

Connection comes from a sense of trust, safety, vulnerability and mutual respect. Being the social creatures that we are, we all crave connection. We all want to belong, to feel seen, heard and appreciated by another human being. I think you can probably agree that connection is a vital part of life. Do you know, however, what connection means to you?

Take a moment and close your eyes. Focus on your breath. Take two or three deep breaths: inhale through your nose, feel your belly expand, guide your breath up to your heart space, breathe light and energy into your heart, then breathe out. Stay here for a moment and reflect on the word 'connection'. Bring up a memory of deep connection in your life: where you truly felt seen, accepted, heard. You would've given anything to stay there forever. Where were you? What were you doing? Who else is in this picture? What made your connection so strong?

You probably saw yourself sitting close to someone. Some sort of display of affection was probably involved. Maybe you were holding hands, or wrapped in a warm embrace. Most people I've asked say they associate connection with being in someone's physical presence. If that is how we see connection, how do we cultivate it at a distance – such as when extenuating circumstances leave us isolated from our loved ones?

I remember asking my grandparents a similar question several years ago. They were in their mid-eighties, having been together for over 70 years. I was sitting across from them in their study, as my grandfather told jokes and my grandmother, who would rather balance uncomfortably on the arm of his chair than sit in a different seat, laughed lovingly while caressing his hair. I had always admired their fairy tale romance, their deep connection and their undying devotion to each other. I couldn't believe it when they told me the story of the five years they spent apart as young adults, when my grandfather was studying abroad. Phone calls were not easy to come by. Letters took up to a month to arrive; if they arrived at all. Being physically apart from someone was truly limiting, yet somehow their relationship stood the tests of both time and limited communication technology.

We have come a long way from telegrams, donkey deliveries and rotary phones. Most of us can pull a device out of a pocket and within moments hear a familiar voice or see the smiling face of a loved one. Social media, video conferencing and apps have expanded our individual worlds by allowing us to stay in touch with people all over the globe and meet complete strangers who quickly become friends. Yet, despite the ease with which we can reach people, so many of us feel disconnected.

Awareness

One of the foundations of mindful connection is awareness. It comes from paying loving attention to what is going on in the moment, and it involves tuning in to your thoughts and emotions non-judgementally.

The greatest misgiving people express about connecting with others online comes from the misunderstandings that often occur. There is a disconnect that comes from the feeling of being with someone and yet feeling their absence at the same time. While the screen can seem like a barrier, the real barrier to connection is our lack of self-awareness.

When facing adversity, most of us look outside of ourselves for answers. We fall into the media wormhole, looking for solace, while forgetting to shine the flashlight inwards. We feel alone because we have not learned how to be with ourselves in a loving and fulfilling way.

Pause for a moment. Take two or three deep breaths. What do you see, hear, smell, taste and feel right now? Focus on the challenging situation you are experiencing: the impact it is having on the world, your co-workers, your friends, your family and ultimately yourself. Feel into your body: are there any tight spots, any tension you are holding in your shoulders, head, neck or back? What are the thoughts and emotions racing through your mind? How have you been during your interactions with others? What have you been refusing to look at?

People usually have one of two reactions to challenging times: either they enter a state of denial, claiming they are fine while stubbornly shoving all their emotions under the rug; or they allow themselves to fall into a seemingly endless fight/flight state, handing the reins over to fear. Neither of these reactions are a basis for deep connection.

You may ask, what about the people who grow? Well that, my friends, is not a reaction – it is a response. A response is a decision rooted in self-awareness, while a reaction is based on conditioning, or how you have always automatically reacted.

Deep connection requires self-awareness. Often, when faced with adversity, our fears, anxieties and insecurities become heightened. We can easily be triggered and trigger others due to the unconscious impact the situation is having on us. Be aware of how you are showing up. If you schedule a call with someone, let that be the only thing you do during that time. Turn off all distractions and simply be with that person. Listen wholeheartedly, ask them questions, and show them you are interested in what they have to say. Give yourself space before the call to become aware of how you are feeling. Ground yourself and take three deep breaths.

Become aware of where you tend to hide. If you are someone who doesn't like being seen, both metaphorically and physically, I challenge you to step out of your comfort zone. Next time you are on a video call, turn on your camera. Let people see you! While virtual backgrounds are fun to explore, I encourage you not to rely on them. There is something so powerful about inviting others into your physical space. Whenever I see people sitting in their house, I feel like I have had a glimpse into their world and who they are. That may sound scary to some people; however, opening yourself up to that experience allows the other person to feel much closer to you.

I recently attended an online workshop called Moving Connections. The facilitator, Georgia Shine, made a powerful analogy that stuck with me:

"We come together from all over the world; in our bedrooms, our kitchens and living rooms, and share connection through an online portal. The absence of one shared physical space brings about the necessity for a more abstract understanding of the space we share in order to experience cohesion as a group-body. This has led me to imagine that we are each in a petal of one collective flower. The screen represents the attachment of the petal to the circular, pollen-filled centre where we can enliven each other with our discoveries – our poetry, dance and song. As a group, we can decide on the colour, the shape and texture of the whole flower and each individual petal. The metaphor can be enhanced and grown by the reflections of individuals as the session builds. This online flower is a beautiful way to discover the creative opportunity that separation brings, while helping to maintain spatial multidimensionality when interacting with a flat screen."

Sharing what is in your heart in an honest and vulnerable way is key to forming connections. There is, however, a balance that needs to be struck. Be careful not to turn the other person into your sounding board. Be aware of their needs too. Giving them time, while holding the space with compassion, will make them feel seen, heard and, in turn, more connected to you.

Acceptance

Acceptance is the most important attitude in cultivating mindful connection, and yet the most difficult to achieve.

Zoom is a video chat platform many people use to connect with each other. As a life coach and meditation teacher, I spend a lot of time on Zoom. It is my favourite way to connect online, as it's the closest thing to in-person interaction. However, I will admit that it can feel draining after a while. One of the chief complaints from people who are transferring both their professional and social interactions online is something that I call 'Zoom fatigue'. I believe this comes from the cognitive dissonance of feeling someone's presence and absence simultaneously. You are happy to be seeing their face, hearing their voice and interacting, while also wishing you could be with them in person.

If you expect online interactions to be the same as in-person ones, you are resisting the situation rather than allowing it to be as it is. When you accept that this is something completely different, and a whole new way of connecting, you enter a state of flow. You look at the situation with curiosity and enter a state of discovery. For those of us who have resisted technology or social media in the past, embracing the uniqueness of this situation opens a whole new world to us. Instead of feeling overwhelmed by the difficulty of navigating all these different communication tools, we open ourselves up to learning and growing, and come to appreciate all the wonderful aspects that this new experience brings.

Creativity

I have come to understand and appreciate the power of adversity in cultivating creativity. I believe we all have an inner artist lying dormant inside us, waiting to be set free. Many people get stuck in autopilot, following the same routines and having the same experiences and interactions, day in and day out. Suddenly being catapulted out of our comfort zones and forced into new ways of being can be the match that lights our creative fire. Once we stop resisting and start embracing, we begin to explore and find new ways to do the things we love.

With the world in isolation during the coronavirus pandemic, many people have found themselves missing the ways in which they used to interact with others. With everyone desperately seeking connection, it requires creativity to nurture and deepen existing relationships – and to build new ones.

Ask yourself how you can bring the things you love about your normal life into this 'new normal' you are creating. To help get your creative juices flowing, here are some ideas for you and your close connections to try:

- Explore different flavour combinations and connect through your love of food! Cook the same meal, compare dishes and eat them at the same time over a video call. You could even create your own group on social media so you can share recipes, which gives you the benefit of not having to plan every meal – plus, you'll meet new people.
- Teach a friend or family member new skills, or learn something together online, like a language – people who learn together, grow together.
- Watch a favourite film and discuss it. Metaphorically curl up on the couch and share a bowl of popcorn.
- Make videos and share them using apps like Marco Polo.

- Dance or exercise together online. Laugh, move your body and improve your health, while increasing your connection. Become accountability buddies on your journey to better physical fitness!

- Host virtual book clubs, karaoke parties, game/quiz nights and even happy hours using Zoom or apps like Houseparty.

- Hug someone with your eyes. If you're looking for soul-baring connection with others and you're willing to push yourself out of your comfort zone, try a website called Human Online, where you share a minute of eye contact with a complete stranger. I dare you to try it and not cry!

Whatever it is you'd like to do, I guarantee there is an app, a group or some online community doing it. The same goes for any challenging situation you might be in. Look for a Facebook group or online community of like-minded people who are either going through the same thing or have been through it and can support you. And if you don't find a group doing something you want to do, create it! There are bound to be others out there waiting for it.

Remember:

- This time of limited in-person interaction is an opportunity to gain awareness of our internal world, create better connections with ourselves and connect with others in a deeper way. Listen to my connection meditation at TeachMindfulnessOnline.com/book.

- Adversity is a part of life, and when faced with it, we have two options: we let ourselves crumble and pull away from others, or we lean in, we rise and we grow together. We accept the situation, the pain and hardship and, in so doing, embrace all of the positive aspects that come with it.

- You are not alone. At your fingertips, on the other side of a screen, are millions of people who are also going through their own challenges and yearning to connect. Put yourself out there, be loving and compassionate, show up, and you will emerge from this situation stronger, better and, most importantly, together.

About Melissa Acuna-Dengo

Melissa is an inner transformation coach and mindfulness and meditation teacher with a mission to integrate mindfulness into education and help others lead joy-filled, fulfilling lives. She lives in Texas, USA.

https://www.facebook.com/Curiously-Connected-950336991971905/

20

Mindful Ways to Work from Home

Yvonne Cookson

Have you ever experienced working from home while trying to juggle what seems like 1,000 other things? Discipline is required as, without the structure and routine of going to a place of work, we're left to our own devices.

On a good day, working from home can mean productive hours, exercise and healthy meals. But what about those bad days? We can find ourselves raiding the fridge, not leaving the house, staying in our pyjamas, and struggling to find the motivation to keep working.

The challenges we're currently experiencing in this pandemic are putting on hold the need for us to commute, wear smart clothes or put our makeup on. However, many of us will be yearning to go into work, enjoy a coffee and catch up with our colleagues, and experience the structure and routine that a typical working day can give.

Mindfulness can help us manage the difficult moments and also to really appreciate the good times in life. Mindfulness techniques can be a great way to keep us calm, focused and grounded. However, it's not a 'one size fits all' solution, and different approaches and techniques resonate for different people and circumstances.

Mindfulness practices can help to lift our mood and energy levels and keep us feeling connected. In this chapter, I share some tips to help you create a mindful daily routine that works for you and your household during unusual times. I include some insights from people that I've interviewed about their experiences of working from home in more mindful ways. You can also listen to a guided meditation for mental control for working from home at TeachMindfulnessOnline.com/book.

"I'm no longer a manic stress ball. When I was commuting, I was sitting in traffic and missing lunch. I feel calmer and I see so much positivity from this (awful) situation. I'm at home with my dog, who I know won't be with us much longer. I think embracing the stillness will be good for many of us."

Routine, Routine, Routine!

"Get up like you're going to work: shower, breakfast, walk the dog. Put on the washing or do the dishes, then sit down and make a plan for what you can achieve today."

A simple routine can make all the difference. Having a structure enables us to be more productive and allows us to sense that reassuring feeling of normality. It also helps to regulate our body clock, which in turn can improve our quality of sleep (Chapter 5 reflects further on managing your sleep during challenging times). Try and get up around the same time every day and start the morning with a good breakfast. This enables us to think with an open and clear mind.

"Routine has been amazing for my mindfulness, and I feel the happiest and most content I've felt for a very long time."

"I've found the best way to 'get ahead' is to get up really early before anyone else is up. I feel like I've already allowed for the distractions I will come across during the day."

Aim to always get dressed in your workwear. Wearing shoes while working from home can also help (we associate wearing slippers with being at home, and we aren't in work mode). Treat your morning routine like you're about to start a 'normal' day at work. This changes your state of mind and puts you into the correct frame of mind to have a productive, happy day.

Without routine, it is extremely easy to get distracted with daily chores, home-schooling, parenting, partners and pets. Many of the people I interviewed stated that routine was needed for them to focus on their mindfulness, but that distractions in the home hindered their productivity and workflow.

"I still stick religiously to my morning routine: this involves exercise, journal writing, task setting, affirmations, reading and mindfulness. It frames my mind and body to be primed for the day, and the right stuff gets done."

"Now I've got myself into a good routine, I'm finding it much easier to switch off from everything else."

Set Boundaries

"I'm lucky to have an office at home, but it isn't easy when there's no structure to the day and I'm not working to tight deadlines, which I now realise I kind of miss."

Boundaries are key – they give us structure, security and help us with our routines. A tidy house and workspace help to create a tidy mind and enhance a sense of tranquillity. Always try to make the beds, keep the living areas tidy, and open the curtains to give natural light to each room. Notice how keeping living areas tidy can clear your mind, ready for a productive day.

Aim to have a designated workspace within your home where possible, and try to work to set times. This can help you keep a clear focus on what you need to do that day.

"The first few weeks I found it hard due to distractions. Also, my office is my dining table, which is not ideal! I also constantly have the urge to get up and put a wash on, hang it out and clean the house!"

"I've changed my spare room into a dance studio to film my classes, and from a mindful perspective it really makes me feel like I'm coaching within a studio. I now feel more prepared for these classes than when I wasn't working from home and I was doing 14-hour days."

"I try to get up at a normal time (with a cheeky lie-in every now and again). I break for lunch – something I never had time to do

before – and I finish at 4 p.m., shut the laptop lid and don't go back to it. I don't kick myself if I break off to watch a film with my kids or sit in the sun for an hour."

It is also extremely important that we don't beat ourselves up when we have had a bad day. We should all allow for this every now and again. After all, we're only human and we're living through some extreme challenges. Never forget that it's okay not to feel okay – remember to always be kind to yourself. We need to allow these feelings to sit with us, accept them and let them pass.

Treat your weekends and downtime differently, so you don't get into the habit of allowing the days to roll into one. Remember to differentiate between work and leisure times. When you've finished your working day, put away the tools of your trade, such as your laptop, computer and books, and take some time to relax in the evening before the routine starts again the following day.

"I don't sit in my living room at all until after 6 p.m. or watch TV in the day, so it still feels like an evening luxury."

"We make sure we put all work out of sight for the weekend."

Moving, Moments and Meditation

"I'm doing yoga every morning, and we all go for a walk after the last conference call of the day. I also take a walk in the garden every time I have a cuppa."

When our minds feel full or we are worrying, it helps to think about what we're able to control and try to come back to the present moment. Be gentle and kind with yourself, and use healthy distractions to overcome any negative feelings.

Movement is just as important for your mind and your mental state as it is for your body. Taking regular breaks to move around can help make the day pass more quickly. Gentle stretches can help release tension; walking up and down in your living room or walking around the garden can help get the blood and endorphins pumping; and a lively dance session can be a great way to improve your mood, as well as burning some calories! Read Chapter 9 and enjoy some mindful yoga. If possible, try to go outside daily and enjoy being in nature. If this isn't an option, try to find a view outside from your working area, as this can help you feel grounded.

Try to give yourself some relaxing practices every day to help maintain your wellbeing. Try a quick hand massage, a short breathing meditation or just listening to some music to calm your mind. Keeping yourself well hydrated and full will also help you to think straight.

Slowing down your breathing can also help calm your mind and body, but if focusing on just the breath feels challenging, try to move with the breath instead. Short breathing meditations are a perfect way to practise throughout the day (choose one from the audio tracks at TeachMindfulnessOnline.com/book). Start by resting with your hands palms up. As you breathe in, open your hands, and as you breathe out, make a gentle fist. Try to focus on moving your hands and notice how this relaxes your breathing and makes you feel centred. This exercise is a great diversion from an overflowing mind.

"I have taken webinar opportunities on wellbeing when time permits."

"It is important to accept this is a different way to work and embrace all the aspects of it. Breathe in between tasks and focus on what you can control, as well as allowing for self-care."

Reach Out

"I'm keeping in touch with the office staff and checking in with them, because it's harder than you think when you're used to seeing someone every day."

Keeping in touch with colleagues is vital, as working from home can be lonely and isolating. Make the time to connect with others by talking on the phone, sending text messages and, more importantly, having regular video calls. By making time to see fellow workers on screen you can keep your relationships more personal and real, which is far more effective than just hearing a voice at the end of a phone.

"I'm managing to keep in touch with colleagues via email and our chat room. I do miss face-to-face contact though."

Be Grateful, and Be Kind to Yourself

"I find this both physically and mentally exhausting – it seems to take a different sort of energy. I've doubled my meditation time in the morning, but I haven't quite cracked the evenings yet and I constantly feel tired."

No one knows all the answers during this challenging time. Our emotions are highly sensitive and heightened as we feel fearful, confused and have no idea of when the current situation is going to end. However, these challenges will end at some point, and we should try our hardest to hold onto a positive mindset.

Take each day as it comes and use your 'reset' button each night. Live in the now and try to cultivate a 'gratitude attitude', even on the bad days (which we all have). Practising gratitude and journalling is a great way to help you feel better during challenging circumstances. Research shows that writing down what we feel grateful for every day increases our happiness and reduces depression. Give it a try for a week to see if it works for you, and check out Chapter 12 for more on gratitude.

You may decide to utilise your time to do something you've never found time for before, like taking up a new hobby or interest – but genuine downtime is important too. In the same way that you switch off your phone and computer, remember to make time to 'switch off' and nurture yourself. Mindful choices include reading books, practising yoga, meditating, watching TV programmes and films that inspire you, listening to music that you love, or trying your hand at journalling.

"To inspire and entertain others, I've released my books on Facebook for families to read. I've also created colouring books for those who can't draw but like to colour in. Don't give up, get a creative plan!"

"We're just embracing the positives of working from home, such as no commute, saving money, time with our dog and lovely mindful walks."

"I finish off the day with a walk. It's like walking home from work, giving me time to switch off."

Remember:

- Some of these mindful techniques may not be 'the norm' for a typical working environment, but they may help you positively adjust to and cope with the challenges of your new-look working day.
- Try not to be too hard on yourself: practise self-kindness and aim to accept the not-so-good days as well as the good ones.
- We spend a huge part of our lives working – we might as well be mindful, kindful and grateful while we do it!

About Yvonne Cookson

Yvonne is a mindfulness teacher and holistic therapist. She believes that mindfulness has changed her life, and now she wants to help change the lives of others for the better. She lives in Harrogate, UK.

www.serenitawellness.co.uk

21

Staying Mindful with Difficult People

Shabbir Ahmed and Shraddha Shah

One day, two sparrows were enjoying the rain from their nest. A monkey came to take shelter under the same tree, drenched and shivering. One of the sparrows came out and said, "You wouldn't suffer like this if you had built a home like us. If we can create a nest with small beaks, why can't you with two hands and two legs?"

The monkey was not in a good mood, and asked the sparrow to shut up.

The sparrow continued, explaining how much effort they'd taken, and how they didn't suffer from any bad weather conditions.

As the sparrow kept giving its advice, the monkey climbed up and destroyed the nest in frustration.

We may be able to relate to one of the characters in the story. Perhaps a spouse, family member or relative may act like the sparrow or monkey.

Four Friends

When we were invited to write on this topic, we decided to interview four friends who had dealt with difficult people (a spouse, in-laws, parents or kids) within the family – people who were the source of much frustration in their life. They wished they could change that other person, and disliked how they behaved or spoke.

A difficult person is someone whose behaviour you believe often creates challenging emotions and feelings within you. Life doesn't always allow you to stay away from such people, and it provides plenty of situations that can trigger sparrow and monkey behaviour!

The journey of life has exposed these four friends to transformative learning and mindfulness skills, and they have realised that the only person they have control over and can change in the world is themselves, and no one else.

Here is what helped them:

- **Friend 1:** "I am more aware now, and I consider my response to the other person. The grip of living in the past has lessened, and I don't bring the past into conversations. Now, I become aware of my emotions quickly and don't get carried away like a speeding car, which was the case earlier. Though I was always empathetic, I now have more clarity on when I am biased or judging."

- **Friend 2:** "I pay careful attention now, which gives clarity. Not reacting immediately and allowing the other person to complete expressing their views is helping me in my dealings with them. I'm willing to understand others' perspectives, accepting what makes sense – sometimes we are wrong and only attached to our point of view. Awareness and responding accordingly is the key."

- **Friend 3:** "The assumption that my in-laws were criticising me and my relationship with my spouse was wrong, and was the cause of the whole war in my head. Being aware of these thoughts gave me relief. I have become cheerful again!"

- **Friend 4:** "You have to be in listening mode even with a difficult person, and not immediately reacting. Give input only when others are interested. Every person has a limit: identify yours, and avoid situations that may trigger you."

Automatic Thoughts versus Thinking

Our minds are often wandering in autopilot mode, rather than present and conscious in the here and now. For example, imagine if, while driving your car, the automatic thought pops up in your head with the question, "What shall I do this weekend?" You unconsciously start planning your weekend, only to realise later that your mind has drifted, at which point you bring it back to the present (driving). Not much later, this might happen again; you may notice, or maybe not.

The average person thinks tens of thousands of automatic thoughts per day. Unfortunately, the majority of those thoughts are negative.

There are various categories of negative automatic thoughts, such as:

- Mind-reading ("He wants to change me")
- Assuming ("She is making fun of me")
- Blaming ("He never misses the opportunity to criticise me")
- All or nothing ("I feel so helpless")
- Fortune-telling ("My future is bleak")
- Catastrophising ("My life is a mess")
- Comparing ("I wish I were someone else")
- Not accepting ("I can't stand this anymore")
- False beliefs ("I can change them")

The good news is that you are not your thoughts! This might be surprising to many. You have no control over what thoughts should pop up inside your head. However, if you are aware, you can choose how to respond to an automatic thought in a better way. You can give it space, so it arises and passes by.

As Martin Luther once said, "You cannot keep birds from flying over your head but you can keep them from building a nest in your hair."

Now, you can look at the automatic thought examples above and can guess what automatic thoughts monkeys or sparrows (or others around you) might have, which make them feel the way they do and so act accordingly.

Being Mindful of Thoughts, Feelings and Actions: Going beyond Positive Thinking

Imagine it's the rainy season and your son is going out to buy medicine for you. You asked him to carry an umbrella, but he ignored you as it's not raining yet.

Now an hour has passed: he hasn't returned, it is raining heavily outside now, and you realise he forgot to take his phone. What thoughts do you have? Take a moment to think about this before reading further.

Some of the responses may be:
- He never listens; he didn't take an umbrella.
- He just does what he wants to do.
- Because of him, I won't be able to take my medicine on time.
- He will be angry when he gets back, as I sent him to buy medicine and he'll be soaked.
- Let me step out and see where he is; an hour has passed.
- He will be back when the rain settles down.
- I hope he is well, he forgot his phone as well.

Now, based on what you thought (perhaps a negative automatic thought), you will feel emotions, and then you will act accordingly. For example:

1. If you thought "I hope he is well", you will feel concerned (fear or sadness), and your action will be extra care and love when he returns.
2. If you thought "He never listens", then you will feel frustrated (anger), and your action will be to tell him off or ignore him (or something similar) when he arrives.

If negative automatic thoughts popped up, you might start building further negative thinking on top of it and then feel and act accordingly. Whereas, if you are aware, you have the choice of dealing with automatic thoughts so you can feel better and act wisely.

Some people think the solution to these negative automatic thoughts is to try thinking more rationally or positively. However, taking a mindful approach is different. Instead, the idea is to just see these thoughts as thoughts. Then, you can step back and refocus on whatever you need to do next. Fighting your thoughts is not the solution.

Strong emotions weaken over time. Even the strongest feelings produced due to cravings may be diluted within 15–20 minutes. If the monkey had known this, he might have waited, acknowledging the strength of his emotions, or he might have removed himself from the situation instead of destroying the sparrows' nest.

Every incident will generate some automatic thoughts (maybe negative), that might not be reality. How you feel and act is not due to the situation or person but because you believe your thoughts to be true.

Changing your relationship to your thoughts will help you to manage your thoughts more effectively and stay mindful when you are with a difficult person.

Dealing Mindfully with Difficult People

Being aware of automatic thoughts needs practice, like any other skill – as does being aware of your feelings and actions. If we are not aware of these thoughts, we will "get carried away like a speeding car" (as one of the friends we interviewed said).

The same is true for the difficult people we have to deal with, yet they might not have these skills. Their actions, what they feel, might be based on the automatic thoughts they have. We're not saying that this justifies a difficult person's actions, but it helps to understand how automatic thoughts fuel incidents – we can act wisely when we're more aware of our thoughts.

If we're in a similar situation as the sparrow, we may be aware of when to give advice and when to keep quiet. If we're in the place of the monkey, we may understand that the frustration we experience is not because of what the sparrow is saying, but our belief in our thoughts about it.

Try to *connect* with people rather than remaining in the grip of your automatic thoughts (which may impel you to want to control the actions of the people around you or the situation you find yourself in). We're not suggesting you need to stay in the company of difficult people who trouble you (if you can help it). However, being aware will help you to see things clearly and not through the various filters of your automatic thoughts, which give a distorted view of reality.

Running away from a difficult person might look like a solution, only for you to realise later that this solution has become another problem for you to solve. Difficult people are everywhere; we can't run away. Bad incidents (with a difficult person) are often situational, but our thoughts replay them – and if we're unaware, this can lead to emotions and actions that further damage the relationship. If this happens on both sides, then it leads to a toxic relationship.

If we become mindful, perceptions can change over time, and the bond with the difficult person can improve.

Here are some tips for staying mindful with difficult people. Take your time to reflect on each point, while you bring to mind a difficult person:

- Don't take personally, or give meaning to, a situation or what someone has said.
- Do a short mindfulness meditation before having a conversation with a difficult person, and after a tough conversation.
- Listen mindfully, being aware of filters/thoughts (judgements, assumptions, interpretations and so on). Don't expect these filters to go away, and be aware that they are just your thoughts (sounds and images popping up in your head).
- What you say is important, but how you say it matters a lot, so be aware of your tone of voice. In certain situations, silence is like a huge noise and can cause others to feel anger. Equally, don't attach meaning to the silence and tone of others.
- Powerful questions can give some space to help a difficult person to be introspective and become aware of their

thoughts, emotions and actions. Don't try to 'fix' them, but do question them mindfully.

- Understand others' perspectives and your bias (watch your thoughts and validate them with reality).
- Think about the difficult person in context, considering all the influences on them. Some actions or words are situational. Like yours, others' thoughts sometimes overpower them to take impulsive action.
- Most of the time, difficult people are suffering in ways that others may not be aware of. Keeping an attitude of compassion and listening mindfully does help in getting to know the reasons behind their actions. Most importantly, choose your timing and listen as if you are listening to the person for the first time.
- Revisit your intention and the broader context of why you are staying with and dealing with this person. Also, give space to consider the other person's intentions as well. Not everyone knows how to express themselves, and they might be coming from the context of concern.

Remember:

- The only person in the world you have control over and can change is you.
- A difficult person cannot destroy your inner peace, but believing your thoughts about the person or situation can. Seeing your thoughts as just thoughts is a mindful solution.
- Mindfulness grows with practice, and your skills of dealing with difficult people improve as you become more aware.

About Shabbir Ahmed and Shraddha Shah

Shabbir Ahmed and Shraddha Shah are accredited life coaches and mindfulness teachers based in Mumbai, India. They strongly believe that mindfulness has many health benefits and can change people's lives.

www.shepherdsinmumbai.com

22

Mindful Ways through Conflict

Tosh Brittan

Conflict is part of being human. It does not come from the peaceful, loving part of us (the part that wants to avoid the conversations we need to have sometimes, or to live without arguments); instead, conflict comes from the innate part of us that gives us the confidence to stand up for what we feel is right and good, and the confidence to be heard and seen.

Conflict is alive in every level of society and in our relationships. So, how do we go about facing and managing those conflictual people, and the places where we sometimes fear to tread? In this chapter, I offer some tips for managing conflict during difficult times by taking a more mindful approach.

Be Accepting

In mindfulness, we talk about accepting and letting go – but this doesn't mean that we allow ourselves to be walked all over by others who are intent on upsetting or hurting us. When we practise acceptance, we begin to understand that there may be other factors unknown to us – ones that affect the person's behaviour and decisions, causing them to act in hurtful ways.

It is good to remind yourself regularly that you cannot control what others say or do, but you always have a choice about how you show up, communicate and act.

For example, your partner may have had a difficult day with the pressures of work. Perhaps they worked through lunch on a call, so they're feeling what many children call 'hangry'! You may be fortunate that your partner is self-aware and tells you that they had a bad day at work; however, they may still be caught up in thoughts about their day and not be aware of their actions, the tone of their voice or whether or not they are present. This is fertile ground for conflict, especially if you too have had a challenging day, or you have financial or self-confidence worries.

It is at times like these that a mindfulness or meditation practice can help you notice the choice you have: to go into conflict, or to come back to a wiser, calmer space (a 'buffer zone' of sorts). The second option allows you to let go, choose your battles and make wiser decisions. It is a place to take a deep breath and reset those monkey-mind thoughts (the ones that race around your mind, demanding that you take action and are heard too).

In the present moment, you are aware that your partner is grumpy, perhaps short-tempered, but rather than resigning yourself to the potential for conflict, you can see clearly that there will be a better time to talk to them later. Instead, practise self-care; so you might take a bath or shower, go for a walk outside, or sit quietly somewhere to meditate, reflect and write down your thoughts before you sleep.

Self-care during conflict is a kindness we do have control over, and even giving yourself a few moments to calm the 'mind monkeys' and their over-catastrophising ways can allow you some space to breathe. This can be as simple as taking a few deep breaths down into your belly before a difficult meeting or before you walk through the door after a stressful day.

Conflict in the Body

Our bodies are a wonderful barometer of how we feel when we are in conflict – whether it is with others or with our own thoughts. The next time you experience conflict in your life, notice how your body is feeling: where in your body do you feel stress, anger or fear? It may be in your stomach – that feeling of being punched in the gut if someone is unkind to you – or it may be the feeling that you have the world on your shoulders as you manage the challenges in your life. Your head may hurt as it is filled with unhelpful thoughts, or your breathing may become shallow when you're feeling stressed and your body is demanding that you find some space to breathe. You can then use these signs to remind you to step back and respond with rest, exercise or a mindful meditation.

Check in with Your Feelings Using HALT

I love the HALT acronym (practised by Dr Christopher Willard), which is useful to reflect on during times of conflict: **Hungry,**

Angry, Lonely, Tired (I add 'Ill', having taught people with chronic disease). If you are going through conflict, whether in a relationship or at work, try checking in regularly with how you are feeling – is it any of these? And if you are feeling any of the elements in HALT (or indeed HALTI), is the person you are in conflict with feeling these things too? It is such a useful reminder, and as you become more aware of your own tiredness, for example, you can make better decisions as to how you manage your day, your commitments and your energy levels.

If you're feeling lonely, being able to gently and kindly communicate this by having the courage to be vulnerable may be helpful. Being open and accepting of how you are feeling, choosing to be brave and reaching out for help not only increases your resilience but is a powerful way to give others the opportunity to help and support you. By understanding how others are feeling, you may be able to practise a little forgiveness, understanding or kindfulness based on how you yourself feel when you're also feeling the same way.

So much conflict happens due to a lack of communication. It is in the power of the words we use that we find connection (or disconnection) with each other. The choice and present-moment awareness to choose the right words is where the real magic happens. Mindful communication is a gift (Chapter 18 delves deeper into mindful communication).

Be Curious about Conflict

Be curious about the triggers that bring conflict into your life. On those days where you feel that nothing is going right, ask yourself – what is it about this day? Taking yourself off automatic pilot can give you valuable information as to when the domino effect of conflict began in your day. It could be the moment your alarm clock didn't go off; it could have been because the children took longer than usual to get ready; or it might be that you've forgotten to allow yourself the time to practise mindfulness (though remember that even a couple of minutes brushing your teeth with your non-dominant hand can be a quick mindfulness practice on a busy morning). You spend the rest of the day playing catch-up.

What can you do to manage the conflict in your life? What areas keep coming up that are challenging, difficult and not working well for you? What can you do differently? It may be something like changing your diet to include fewer stimulants (like coffee or sugary drinks), eating healthier foods, exercising more, reducing social media time or seeing less of those 'energy vampire' friends that drain you: the possibilities are endless.

Soothe the Conflict Within

We often feel conflicted within ourselves. Regret, disappointment and anger can sit inside us for years. For example, when we meet people who divorced many years ago and still feel angry about what happened, we can sense the conflict that resides within them. This brings us back to the choice we have about whether to enter conflict and allow it to become part of our everyday life. Ask yourself: Do I need this on top of everything else? Is it helpful to bear a grudge?

A wise quote comes to mind: "In life, we can't always control the first arrow. However, the second arrow is our reaction to the first. This second arrow is optional." We all have a choice about how we react. We also have the choice to practise forgiveness, even when we feel wronged. By letting go, being the bigger person and leaving our ego at the door, we create a space for the conflict in our lives to drop away.

I remember being on a business trip in Jakarta, Indonesia, in the late 1990s. There was high inflation, civil unrest and conflict. One day, after much shooting and fighting in the streets, the rioters met with a wall of police in full body armour outside the main city gas building, near the police headquarters. As bystanders, we held our breath and watched humanity in conflict at its most challenged – in fight mode. If the gas building caught fire during the riot, we would all die. So we waited, the air thick with hope. A police motorcyclist suddenly drove out from the riot shields towards the rioters. It was in that moment that a choice was made – to continue fighting or to make peace and resolve the conflict by finding a space of kindness, understanding and love. The policeman put out his hand to shake a rioter's hand. It was eagerly taken, the rioter climbed on the back of the bike, and they both drove into the huge crowd, waving and shaking hands, while people clapped and cheered. I shall never forget that incredible scene. We all have a choice in conflict; practising mindfulness helps bring us back to this.

Mindfully navigating your way through conflict involves practising awareness with how you communicate and act. Come back to your breath whenever you're feeling overwhelmed, and remember that you always have a choice about whether or not to enter conflict.

I share a short-guided meditation at TeachMindfulnessOnline.com/book that you may find helpful when managing conflict and trying to find more mindful ways through the experience.

Remember:

- A balanced, kind and supportive group of friends or family members can listen to your concerns and give you non-judgemental and positive advice. Take a step back from any friends, work colleagues or family members who focus on the drama and negative elements that fuel the 'conflict fire'.

- Develop a practice of self-care that includes time for you to be with your most challenging thoughts. This could be through painting, meditating or writing down your thoughts or. Getting our thoughts down on paper gets them out of our heads, giving us all-important head space.

- Take a moment to centre yourself with deep breaths before you attend difficult meetings or spend time with the person you are in conflict with. Sleep on a challenging email or message you need to send rather than instantly reacting, in case you regret your actions later. Ask yourself: What do I realistically want out of this? How will my actions affect the outcome if they are made when I'm stressed, angry or under pressure?

About Tosh Brittan

Tosh is a mindful divorce coach and the founder of Divorce Goddess. She is a podcaster and blogger and has been featured on national TV and in the press. She lives in Surrey, UK.

www.divorcegoddess.com

23

Parenting Mindfully through Challenges

Crysal Olds

"Mindful parenting is the hardest job on the planet, but it's also one that has the potential for the deepest kinds of satisfactions over the life span, and the greatest feelings of interconnectedness and community and belonging." Jon Kabat-Zinn

Mindful parenting is a way of parenting with boundaries in place to protect and contain both yourself and your child(ren) while looking at behaviours, thoughts and experiences with a sense of curiosity, respect, acceptance, compassion and non-judgement, for both yourself and your child. At the same time you remain aware of your own process and trust your child's process. It is a way of life – an underlying energy influencing every decision, action and inaction – and it requires a conscious choice.

Mindful parenting during challenging times can be tough, even for seasoned mindful parents, as, when our own equilibrium is off, it affects everyone around us. It can be extremely hard to support others when you also need support. At times like this it can be easy for us to react instead of responding to behaviours from the children and other adults around us, as we go back to 'default' mode (our parents' parenting style), while our regular rhythm is under review. During this time, we all need increased support in the form of compassion, love and non-judgement from ourselves and others, as we navigate our way through our own process, finding our new rhythm in the sea of uncertainty – effectively needing to parent ourselves while parenting our children.

With mindfulness, we can practise finding a new rhythm through a sense of noticing or awareness of what is, gaining knowledge around what is happening through curiosity, then allowing events to unfold with compassion and non-judgement, without becoming attached to any particular ideas or stories of what that might mean for us. Then we accept. We accept what is with an energy of love, compassion and kindness that we generate within ourselves. Accepting does not always mean that we agree with what is happening or that we enjoy it. It simply means that we accept what we cannot change, and for those areas we can change, we accept our responsibility. Accepting is not really an act of doing, it is a continuance of *allowing* – a softening, an unfurling, a trusting, a sense that we will be okay, even when things are not going the way we desire.

Let's take a look at mindful parenting during challenging times in more detail.

Noticing/Awareness

A challenge can be anything from a child being unable to find the outfit they want to wear to a big change in circumstances – moving to a new house, a new spouse/divorce, being in lockdown due to a virus outbreak... The challenge is in the eye of the beholder. Being aware of how we and our children are experiencing a challenge is a great place to start, and we can do this by regularly noticing. We may notice changes in our or our child's behaviour, tone of voice, needs, body language, body sensations and thoughts that give us a hint that something is challenging for them or us. During big changes in circumstances, try setting a reminder at times throughout the day to just sit and watch your children and yourself with curiosity to get an insight into how they and you are coping. Any changes could be down to exhibiting coping strategies. There is no right or wrong way of coping, it is just a way for us to 'do' something about our situation.

Being curious about our and our children's ways of coping can give insight to our (and our children's) thoughts and actions. This can increase our self-compassion, compassion and non-judgement for 'out-of-character' behaviour that might unfold. This is not to say that regular boundaries should be overlooked (such as not hurting one another), but the ensuing discussion after a breach should be completed with love and compassion and an underlying understanding of why this behaviour developed in the first place. So, it seemed as if Anna hit Ben for no reason at all; in reality, Anna hit Ben because Anna was feeling overwhelmed and Ben got too close – Anna needed more space and didn't know how to verbalise that. This reaction is not age-specific – older children may lash out verbally instead. In the next section, you'll see that this lashing out is a form of 'confrontive coping'.

Ways of coping

Notice which ways of coping you and your children are currently exhibiting (adapted from the Ways of Coping Scale, which you can find more about online):

- Accepting responsibility – acknowledging and accepting the part you played.
- Confrontive coping – standing up for what you believe in; confronting those in power.
- Denial – continuing as normal.
- Escapism – wishing things were different to what they are; trying to feel better through drinking, eating or taking drugs; avoiding others; more screen time; more reading.
- Positive re-evaluation – rediscovering what is important in life; experiencing personal growth/renewed faith.
- Problem solving – generating extra energy to make things work; focusing on a solution.
- Regression – acting from a childlike place or a place of lesser maturity than normal; wanting nurturing; becoming fearful; needing help for things you would ordinarily do by yourself.
- Self-control – going inwards and keeping things to yourself; controlling what you show/tell others.
- Social support – gaining support from others to glean more information or discuss your experience.

Ways of coping may be different for different experiences. So when I face a small stress like not having my normal brand of cereal at the supermarket, I may take the 'positive re-evaluation' view and see it as an opportunity to try a new cereal. Whereas if I was already stressed before going to the supermarket, my coping response may be 'confrontive coping', perhaps having a go at a staff member for not having my cereal in stock.

Exploration

Take some time to sit with the way of coping you feel aligned to now. Close your eyes or soften your gaze. Notice what is happening within your body. Be curious about how this way of coping manifests itself within your body. Notice areas of tension, pain, discomfort, holding; notice areas of ease, spaciousness, expansion, and be curious. Then, turn your attention to your thoughts. What thoughts does this way of coping ignite within you? Just watch and notice them with curiosity.

Now, sit with the way of coping you have identified for each of your children in the same manner. What do you notice?

Allowing

"If you push against nothing, everything that is beneficial will flow easily into your experience." Abraham Hicks

Once we are aware of what we and our children are experiencing, we can move into *allowing*. Allowing requires a sense of trust and faith that each person is capable. With children, this can be hard to fathom because often we take the role of being responsible for our children. Our role is to gently guide and trust that they know their own self and, if not, give them an opportunity to get to know themselves through allowing their experience to unfold naturally, with guidance.

When you notice conflict, question if there is an area where there is a lack of allowing. This can often be thoughts that 'things need to be a certain way'.

At the time of writing, much of the western world was in lockdown due to the coronavirus. My husband, two girls – aged three and six – and I were suddenly living in each other's pockets. My husband and I started this challenge with problem solving and positive re-evaluation coping strategies, as we prepared for weeks of no work and therefore limited income, yet feeling positive about this gift of concentrated family time. The girls delved into a state of distancing and escapism as they continued playing their normal games together and enjoying time to themselves while playing. As time went on, social support came in. We all missed our connections with our friends and extended family, so we created ways around this by scheduling video calls and making cards to send. Confrontive coping then came in as each of our coping strategies clashed – self-control and regression – we denied allowing each other and ourselves to just be and focused on the negative rather than the positive. The girls started needing help with things they had been doing for themselves for a long time, and their play changed to taking turns being babies. My husband and I were defensive as we expected more from each other than each could give.

After a couple of days in this space, there was an awakening as I moved into accepting responsibility. I accepted responsibility that I needed to start *allowing* (resting when I needed to, working only when I was inspired, completing projects when feeling creative), and acknowledging to my girls I hadn't been there for them, like I normally am, because I was having a tough time coping too. They replied with hands on my shoulder and an "it's okay, Mum". Moving into this phase changed all of our coping strategies. When one person is low, the whole group experiences it; likewise, when one person rises, the whole group rises.

When we rest and relax (or simply allow, physically and mentally), we enable a reconnection with our true selves and with each other. This reconnection gives us the opportunity to reflect and re-evaluate and move forward mindfully.

Being mindful when boundaries are breached

Allowing is not an opportunity for boundaries to be breached. If the outcome is a breach of a boundary (such as your children hurting each other), then a mindful conversation with those involved (one-on-one, in private) is required.

I share a meditation on responding with compassion that you might like to try before you engage: visit TeachMindfulnessOnline.com/book.

Here's how to have a mindful conversation (adapted from *How to Be the Parent You Always Wanted to Be* by Adele Faber and Elaine Mazlish):

- Develop a connection – express gratitude for something they did, engage with them on a current project.
- Discuss what you have noticed – stick to the facts, not conjecture: "I noticed that you really hurt Ben."
- Show understanding: "This is not normally like you, and I understand things are hard at the moment and we all deal with that in different ways."
- Invite their point of view: "How are you feeling about hurting Ben?"

- Respond through mindfully listening and communicating your interpretation of their view. Continue this process until they feel understood/heard. You may see this in their body as a release/softening or through eye contact/connection, or they may verbally tell you.

- Briefly discuss your view: "I felt sad when you hurt your brother. I am here to help keep you and Ben safe. Is there a way you would like me to help you with that?"

- Join forces to find a resolution. Perhaps they need things from you/others in the situation. You may need to start out with a few ideas: "How can we help you get the space you need when you are feeling overwhelmed?"

- Non-judgementally note down all ideas: "Have Ben move out"; "Spend time outside by myself"; "I let you know I need help with a scream/calling your name"; "You take Ben with you so I can release the emotion safely."

- Mutually decide on a way forward: "Great, so we agree that when you are feeling overwhelmed you can […], and I can help you by […]."

Acceptance

"Accept – then act. Whatever the present moment contains, accept it as if you had chosen it. Always work with it, not against it. This will miraculously transform your whole life." Eckhart Tolle

You may have days of to-ing and fro-ing, bargaining with the experience (or with the child) to behave the way you desire, which inadvertently encourages a 'digging in of toes'. After you have gained insight into this dance and you begin to allow, you soften, accepting that it is their or your journey. When we approach another with acceptance, the push-back is no longer required. The acceptance you feel of the situation is felt by the other person. You are both then able to move forward with re-connection, reflection and re-evaluation rather than defensiveness.

I share a guided meditation on the path to acceptance that you may like to try: visit TeachMindfulnessOnline.com/book.

During a challenging time, accept that:

- Deep down, no matter what happens, you and your child are, and always will be, okay.
- You are the greatest teacher for your child – even on your worst days. In handling yourself with care, compassion, love and kindness, when you are struggling, you are teaching them a lifelong skill.
- We all need rest and relaxation to reconnect (with ourselves and each other), reflect and then re-evaluate. Allow, and the rest will follow.
- Gaining insight and repairing relationship ruptures through mindful communication (refer to Chapter 18) are what matters. Your acceptance allows others to move forward and enables a re-connection.
- When we focus on the positive, we feel energised. When we focus on the negative, we feel depleted. You have a choice.
- Uninterrupted time between you and your child, where you are truly present, will heal all.

Remember:

- Awareness: Notice your and your child's coping strategies on a regular basis. Be aware that changes in behaviour, tone and body language, body sensations and thoughts are all indicators of ways of coping. Be curious. How is this being experienced? Be aware that coping strategies change.

- Allowing: Refrain from pushing back and welcome an allowing of what is to unfold in its own time, with compassion, love, kindness and non-judgement. If you notice conflict or a 'pushing back', be curious about where there is a lack of allowing.

- Acceptance: Accept that you have a choice of how you respond. Accept with non-judgement and know that in doing so, you allow others the space to accept.

About Crysal Olds

Crysal Olds lives in Nelson, New Zealand, with her husband and two home-schooled children. She has a degree in Psychology and Criminology and is trained in several client-centred holistic therapies, including teaching mindfulness.

www.mindovermatter.co.nz

24

Mindful Co-parenting and Single Parenting

Elspeth Lewis

Parenting as a single parent or as a co-parent (where two or more adults share the responsibility of raising and caring for children together, usually from separate locations) is a challenging enough task in normal times. UK single-parent charity, Gingerbread, notes that twice as many are likely to be living in poverty compared to coupled households. At times of crisis, any pre-existing difficulties are likely to be amplified as emotions run high. However, when co-parenting, it can also be an opportunity for both parties to work together much more effectively in the best interests of the children.

Recognising the Challenges

Single-parenting

If you are single-handedly taking responsibility for your child or children, it is important to begin by recognising and accepting the challenges that you are possibly facing. These may include:

- Lack of physical and moral support
- Potential financial difficulty
- Pressure of having to provide for the family
- Tiredness and exhaustion
- Lack of 'breathing space'
- Feeling the need to be continuously fit and healthy, as the sole carer

In recognising the actual challenges of your situation, you become aware of your starting point and can allow yourself to accept your limitations. Try not to compare your activities and achievements with those of friends with two-parent families.

It is important that we acknowledge when our circumstances are vastly different and know that one situation is not better than the other. Two-parent families have a host of other challenges to navigate!

Co-parenting

One of the biggest challenges you face in co-parenting is re-establishing a new parenting relationship with the other parent, while leaving your previous personal relationship behind.

When you no longer live together, it's impossible to have a 360-degree view of what is happening at the other parent's house. Unless you have a very open co-parenting partnership, you are unlikely to know of issues that may be affecting the other parent's career, health or relationships.

There may be a sense that part of your child's life is completely unknown, and this can generate a sense of loss of control. In a time of crisis, you may also experience concerns for your child's safety.

Responding Mindfully

In this section, I share some tips for responding mindfully to parenting challenges during difficult times. I would also like to share two guided meditations that you may find helpful as a single parent or co-parent: the compassionate pause and a self-compassion practice for challenging times. Visit: TeachMindfulnessOnline.com/book.

Single parenting

If you feel alone and unsupported, it is very commonplace to tell yourself that you are not enough.

You can reduce this suffering by kindly and gently reminding yourself that you are enough and that you are doing the best that you can manage right now.

It is also helpful to remember that there are millions of other single parents around the world, experiencing exactly the same thoughts and feelings. Joining a support group may be helpful, especially one where members share useful tips and ideas.

Learn to recognise when you need to pause and have a rest, even if this is just a three-minute mindful pause or a five-minute cup of tea.

It's also very important to let go of any sense of self-judgement, and to reach out to friends and family when you need help and support.

Co-parenting

Set an intention to put your child's needs first and try not to get drawn in by any negative behaviour from others.

When emotions are running high and someone else's behaviour towards you seems unfair and unjust, feelings such as frustration, irritation and anger can creep in. It's impossible for you to guess what might be going on in the background. You can try to remain open to the possibility that there are stresses and strains behind the behaviour, and to respond mindfully rather than to react defensively.

Responding mindfully may include stepping back from sending an angry, defensive email if you feel provoked, and pausing until you are in a calmer state of mind.

Mindfully co-parenting requires letting go of past patterns of behaviour from your previous relationship and being respectful within the framework of your new co-parenting relationship.

It can take time and a lot of practice, but letting go of any anger and hostility allows you to shift unnecessary emotional weight that may otherwise hold you back.

Co-parenting mindfully – my personal experience

During the coronavirus pandemic, I agreed with my ex-husband that we would change our contact arrangements slightly, as he was no longer able to have our children stay overnight during the week.

Being a real creature of habit (we all like routine!), this filled me with apprehension. What would happen afterwards? I did not want to set a new precedent, whereby I would miss seeing my children every other weekend.

My natural instinct was to resist, as I would miss having that downtime with them during the weekends. I thought my house would be seen as the 'home-schooling' venue and his place the 'house of fun'! However, with me single-handedly home-schooling the children from Monday to Friday, the set-up made practical sense in the interim.

In fact, by the time we got to the weekends, I was so relieved to have some respite and the opportunity to do my own work if I needed to that I was grateful for the break. I built in some downtime with the children during the week too, so that we didn't feel the loss of our weekends together.

The thought of driving the 60-mile round trip to my ex-husband's house felt like a chore. My inner voice would say things like, "Why should I have to make that journey? He moved away, so this is his problem! I can't afford these fuel costs!" However, making the decision to be supportive for the sake of the children not only demonstrated to him that I wanted to work together, but it also showed the children that I was supportive of this arrangement.

In the end, the journey was a welcome break from the monotony of isolating at home with the children. We saw new scenery, we cranked up the radio and had some fun time together out of the house!

My own personal learning from co-parenting during a crisis has been that both parties will likely experience extremes of emotion. This can mean that frictions may increase, and both parents need to work effectively to overcome this. However, it also means that there is a genuine sense of commonality and an intention to support each other, for the benefit of the children.

Coping Techniques for Single Parents and Co-parents in Times of Crisis

While you put the needs of your child at the forefront, you also need to ensure that you get enough rest and restorative time for yourself. Self-care is so important, as you can't pour from an empty cup. We cannot parent effectively if we haven't looked after ourselves first.

Here are some coping strategies for two different types of situation.

When you feel unable to control a stressful situation

In this case, you can choose to either *accept* or *adapt to* the stressor. For example, if you feel stressed that you can't have input in behaviours that happen in the co-parent's household:

- Allow yourself to let go of what you can't control.
- Talk to a friend or family member, or try journalling, in order to express your feelings.
- Take time to slow down and focus on nourishing activities such as gardening and playing or listening to music.
- Let go of grudges – holding on to frustration towards a co-parent will upset you and also your child/children.
- Try to see problems as opportunities.
- Lower your expectations. If you are parenting alone, don't compare yourself to two-parent families.
- Take a step back and think of the 'bigger picture' – will this still be a problem in a year's time?
- Look for the good and practise gratitude (refer to Chapter 12).

When you can control the situation

You can choose to either *alter* or *avoid* the stressor, for example:

- Have the regular structure of a loose routine. Having some kind of routine is helpful to minimise the anxiety felt by all during uncertain times of crisis.
- Say no – set clear boundaries.
- Lower your expectations: don't set unachievable goals for yourself.

- Reduce the amount of time spent on social media and watching the news.
- Delegate! For example, ask a parent or friend to help your child with homework over a video app, so that you can have some time for yourself.

Finally, try and introduce some fun and playfulness in your day, in order to shift the emotional tone in your family and alleviate anxiety in both parents and children.

Stories of Hope and Appreciation

At times of crisis, it's important to look for the good. Our minds will be unsettled as they try to navigate this new territory. We may feel under threat and feel that everything is going wrong, so it's vital that we congratulate ourselves on things that go well (or that didn't go wrong!), as well as noting acts of kindness or events that brought us some joy, no matter how minor. Like the blue sky that is always present somewhere, whatever the weather, there are always good things happening around us, even when we feel otherwise.

I reached out to single parents and co-parents at the time of writing, and the positive parenting events they shared with me included:

- Getting together with their co-parent and child at one house on a weekly basis for a takeaway as a family unit.
- Enjoying connecting with their children via technology, such as FaceTime, while not being able to see them face-to-face.

- Seeing older children acting in a very mature manner, and taking responsibility for themselves.
- Having cuddles with their children on the sofa while watching a film together.
- Sharing food items with the co-parenting household, where the relationship had previously been frictional.
- The ex-partner assisting with DIY jobs at the resident parent's home.

"Keeping a record of positive events can help counter our natural tendency to scan our environment for what is going wrong." Zindel Segal, Mark Williams and John Teasdale (from *Mindfulness-Based Cognitive Therapy for Depression*)

Remember:

- Keep reminding yourself of your intention. As a parent, allow your child's needs to come first. This will help you make decisions whenever you feel a sense of injustice or frustration. Remember – your child's needs include you taking care of yourself!
- Mindfully pay attention. Keep checking in compassionately with your own emotions and be aware of the emotions that may be affecting the behaviour of others.
- Be compassionate towards yourself. Compassion is key! Don't set yourself unrealistic goals; instead, look back on what went well today, what pleasantly surprised you, and what brought you some joy (however minor). Notice when you need a break and reach out for support as many times as you need – you may find it in the most unexpected forms.

About Elspeth Lewis

Elspeth Lewis is a mindfulness coach at Pause to Be, based in Edinburgh, who discovered the powerful benefits of mindfulness following bereavement and divorce.

www.pausetobe.co.uk

25

Mindfulness for Helping Professionals

Karen Whitehead

Are you wondering if you fall into the category of 'helping professionals'? Many of us are helpers, but only some qualify as professionals. However, whether you get paid to help or not, mindfulness can be of value if you spend your time tending to the growth and wellbeing of another person.

Responding to Your Own Thoughts and Feelings

Nurses, doctors, caregivers, hospital staff, psychotherapists, counsellors, therapists (physical, occupational, speech), spiritual/religious guides, teachers, coaches and the like often have an extra layer to their personal desire to help: there may be a professional obligation, governed by rules and ethics.

When you're faced with a crisis or a challenging time, like the coronavirus pandemic, or you have thoughts and feelings about something going on personally, such as an argument with your spouse or a nagging backache, your drive to adhere to your professional obligations, ethics and rules can be in conflict with your present-moment experience. When this happens, it's common to feel a sense of overwhelm, uncertainty or internal chaos.

Think about a time when you had other things on your mind, and you had to see a client or patient. Maybe you were getting ready for a vacation and excited to get through your day, or perhaps you were feeling ill or stressed about something in your personal life. You may have even had strong emotions about your client and their situation. What did you do with your own stuff: those thoughts, feelings and physical sensations – the anger at your spouse, worry about your children, pain from backache, or feelings of deep sadness or fear? If you're like most helping professionals, you stuffed it away, locked it down tight, or convinced yourself that it wasn't important and you didn't have time to deal with it.

As helping professionals, our ethics and roles require us to focus on the patient or client. But it's not always easy to do that. In my counselling practice, I see a lot of women with breast cancer and metastatic disease. If one of them receives life-altering news, it can be difficult to be present to their experience while I am dealing with my own reaction. We're more likely to allow ourselves to experience positive thoughts and emotions in the presence of others than negative ones.

One strategy that I have found beneficial is WAIT: *Why Am I Talking*. Sometimes, being present is about sitting with the silence. Waiting for a moment allows us to take a mindful breath and notice our internal state. Once we acknowledge that there is something going on in there, we can choose to shine the light of our attention on what is in front of us instead of what we feel inside. This small action allows you time to validate your own experience at the time it is happening.

Whether you connect mindfulness to meditation, guided visualisation or breathing, mindfulness involves noticing your experience in the present moment. Helping professionals are constantly noticing what is going on for others. As a business/life coach and psychotherapist, I have been trained to notice what others may be feeling or experiencing. Helping professionals have been trained to monitor physical, mental and emotional changes in the people they help.

Sometimes, this training can result in a lot of self-monitoring. I once worked with a physician who thought she had developed some of the same symptoms as her patient. When she had a headache, she thought it might be a brain tumour, not tension from hours sat at a computer. A new therapist might wonder if he's depressed if he feels unmotivated or sad. But this is different from the type of awareness that comes with mindfulness. Being mindful allows you the opportunity to be curious about a feeling or sensation, so you can recognise that there may be other, more likely explanations for your experience.

The stress that develops from holding back or denying our own experience can lead to depression, anxiety, compassion/empathy fatigue or burnout. The weight can be especially heavy when our internal experience is a traumatic response to what we see every day. During challenging times, it often feels that if we WAIT and take that moment of silence, our own experience may somehow overtake us to the point that we're unable to function in our role. For example, if I allow myself to feel sad and cry, I may never stop. That's a pretty scary thought. Why allow yourself to feel something if you fear it will incapacitate you?

The thing is, once you start acknowledging your own experience by practising mindfulness, you get better and better at choosing where to put your focus. It becomes easier to notice your own grief, anger or fear without being pulled into the crevices of your mind.

How Mindfulness Can Help Us Care for Ourselves

You've probably heard that mindfulness is a good thing. Maybe you've even tried out an app or two, or taken a deep breath when you're stressed. However, if you're anything like I used to be, you may have a laundry list of excuses why you can't or don't have time for mindfulness. For example:

- I can't clear my mind.
- I don't have time.
- It won't work for me.
- I'm too easily distracted.
- I can't sit still.
- I've tried and it didn't work.
- I'll probably do it wrong.

I'm sure you can add to this list. These excuses are about fear: fear that it won't work, fear that it will, fear that someone will judge you. This is what is preventing you from connecting with yourself in a way that can tend to the inner chaos you feel. Once you make the decision that caring for yourself as a caregiver is important and worth your time, you'll begin to see where and how you can be more mindful. Doing something for yourself – investing time and energy in your wellbeing – is difficult for many helping professionals. Helpers, by nature or habit, tend to put everyone else first.

The mindfulness exercises I teach most are ones that can be done quickly and repeatedly throughout the day: between clients, on a lunch break, or before or after work. All you need is a minute or two – less than the time it took you to read that list of excuses! If you love it or begin to see the benefit, you'll find more time.

Practising mindfulness is a way to step back and remind ourselves that we are okay. That moment, hour, or weekend of silence is a reminder to our physiological self that we do not need to be in fight, flight or freeze mode (Chapter 6 goes into more detail about this). As helping professionals, we are exposed to trauma each time we hear or see another human being suffering or in pain. That's the power of shared experience.

Mindfulness helps us to separate our own experience from the people we serve. It helps us to recognise and accept that we are doing all we can in the present moment. The more we practise, the easier it becomes. The more we accept our current situation, the easier it is to think and stay focused on the task at hand. All it means to be mindful is to intentionally notice your present-moment experience with curiosity and acceptance, rather than judgement.

Let's break that down.

- Intention – your mindset; you have a plan to do what you're doing
- Notice – you become aware of your thoughts, emotions or sensations
- Present moment – right here, right now
- Curiosity – showing an interest in
- Acceptance – you acknowledge what you are experiencing (this doesn't mean you like or don't like your experience – that would be judgement!)
- Non-judgement – bring in self-compassion and kindness; be gentle with yourself

You can incorporate these principles in a 30-minute body scan, during a full-day retreat, by moving your body, or by taking some simple diaphragmatic (belly) breaths. I find that including a question helps me be curious rather than judgemental. My favourite question is: *What do I need*? It brings in self-compassion.

Remember, one mindfulness practice isn't better or worse than any other. The one that *resonates* with you is a good place to start. The one you *decide* to do is a good place to start. The one that *feels* good, uncomfortable or scary is a good place to start.

Here are some of my favourite mindful exercises.

1. Take three slow, deep belly breaths. With your first breath, acknowledge what is going on around you. You might hear people nearby, or smell pizza. With your second breath, notice your internal thoughts, feelings and sensations. For instance, *I'm sad about my patient's*

diagnosis, or *My back hurts*. During your third breath, silently ask yourself: *What do I need right now?* You might be surprised by what comes up. (This is a good one to try between patients.)

2. Take a slow, deep belly breath. Thank the universe, your higher power, spiritual guide or another important figure in your life for keeping you safe and grounded. (Try this exercise before your day, before going into work or before seeing a patient.)

3. While washing your hands, wash each finger as if it belongs to someone else. Notice how the water and soap feel and the care that you give. (It may seem silly, but trust me – the resultant self-compassion is amazing!)

4. On the way to work, select a single point of reference on your journey (such as a stop sign, intersection, street sign, doorway). As you head to work, take a deep breath when you see it. At this point, it is time to turn your attention to work or the task at hand. When you see it on your journey home, take a deep breath and turn your attention to home, leaving work behind for the day.

5. Take three to five slow, deep belly breaths as you look around the room. Notice everything that you see. Pay attention to the detail. Think about what it looks like or how it might feel if you touch it.

6. Set a timer for five minutes. Write down the specific thoughts, feelings or sensations that you notice in your mind and body. Write in bullet points, words, phrases – whatever works for you. There is no right way, there is only your way! When the timer goes off, read what you wrote. See if you can separate the facts from the opinions.

7. Sit quietly and think (or write) about all the ways your body and mind have helped you and others. Express gratitude for your gifts. Listen to the short audio track on gratitude at TeachMindfulnessOnline.com/book.

8. Close your eyes and breathe in, visualising a stillness in and around you. As you exhale, notice the difficulty or chaos swirling around you. Breathe in the stillness, breathe out the chaos.

9. Take a regular time each day to check in with yourself. Tie it to something you already do: taking a shower, getting in bed, sitting in the parking lot. This practice can be as short or long as you'd like. Check in with your professional, social, spiritual, emotional and physical self. Notice what bubbles up. Get curious. Ask yourself: *What do I need?* Be gentle with yourself. I share a meditation to guide you through checking in with yourself at TeachMindfulnessOnline.com/book.

10. Start or end your day by closing your eyes and breathing deeply. Acknowledge the fear that keeps you tied up in knots. This might be about your patients or clients, or about yourself and your abilities. Invite it to sit beside you. Get curious about it. Where does it sit in your body? How much space does it take up? When did it start? Notice the separation between you and your fear. Thank your fear for trying to protect you, for trying to keep you safe. With your next breath, feel the strength and courage you have settling between you and your fear. Notice its qualities. Embrace both the courage and the fear. What comes up for you?

As helping professionals, we are at our best when we're taking care of ourselves. "You can't pour from an empty cup," has never been more true in today's society. Our ability to help is directly related to the amount of space and energy we have to dedicate to being present for others.

Mindfulness is a way to create space, to give room to both your experience and the experience of the people you care for. Developing a practice of noticing what is going on internally will allow you to validate and accept your own experience, so you can move through it without stuffing it down or pushing it away.

As a helping professional, you are often very mindful of others' experiences, but not of your own – but you are at your best when you make time to take care of yourself too.

Remember:

- Being non-judgemental can take some practice. Judgement is our way of protecting ourselves. Recognising that we're not in danger in the present moment moves our focus to the facts at hand and allows us to access our gifts for the good of others, while staying grounded in our own experience.
- You CAN put the excuses aside and decide to care for yourself. The intention – choosing to care for yourself – is all you need to get started.
- Start small – include some simple and quick mindful activities you can easily incorporate into your day. As you start to feel the benefits, you can expand your practice.

About Karen Whitehead

Karen Whitehead, LCSW, is a coach, psychotherapist and dog lover who helps women stop the people-pleasing that keeps them overworked and overwhelmed so they can work less and live more! She is based in Atlanta, GA, USA.

www.karenwhiteheadcoaching.com

www.karenwhiteheadcounseling.com

26

Mindfulness for Empathy Fatigue

Michelle Alberigi McKenzie

"Taking care of myself doesn't mean 'me first', it means 'me too'!" L.R. Knost

The other night on the news, I watched as a nurse recorded himself on his phone, crying. He described holding phones for his dying patients so they could talk to their families one last time. People were dying without their families, and families were losing their loved ones without being able to say goodbye.

As I watched this man who was torn apart because he just couldn't do enough to help his patients, I started to cry too. It felt like the world was facing an apocalypse.

The worldwide pandemic has everyone trying so hard to stay safe, and to keep the people they love secure and healthy. Many people are working with these virus victims for long hours, day after day, because there aren't enough qualified people available to help the sick. And they work without the supplies they need to keep themselves safe while helping their patients. These workers are finding themselves running on empty!

Most of us want to live a peaceful life. While it may seem like an impossible task, particularly right now, there are things we can do that may help us achieve a calmer, more serene life.

What's the Difference between Sympathy, Empathy and Compassion?

First of all, let's clarify the difference between how we define sympathy, empathy and compassion. *Sympathy* is when you notice someone else is suffering, but you don't feel it yourself. If I'm sad, and you have sympathy for me, you notice my feeling, but you don't feel it yourself.

***Empathy* is our ability** to sense other people's emotions, coupled with the ability to imagine what someone else might be thinking or feeling. Empathy is the ability to not only understand another's feelings, but also to become one with that person's distress; to put yourself in their shoes and imagine what they're going through in that situation. Empathy is when you feel whatever the other person is feeling. If I'm sad, and you have empathy for me, you feel sad too. Empathy is a good quality, but when we go overboard with it, we suffer.

Compassion is different. *Compassion* is a motivation rather than a feeling. When I'm sad and you have compassion for me, you feel my sadness (empathy) and you're immediately motivated to help in some way, if you can. And if you can't help physically, you have a wish for that suffering to end. With compassion there is also a sense of separation. You realise that I'm sad, but you're not swept up in the feeling. Compassion offers resilience, hope and connection.

Understanding Empathy Fatigue and How to Combat It

Burnout in the helping professions is caused by empathy, rather than compassion. Seeing patients in distress, for example, often makes those caring for them feel distressed too. So although you may hear about 'compassion fatigue', it should be called 'empathy fatigue'.

Matthieu Ricard, the French translator for the Dalai Lama (who is involved in research in the areas of empathy and compassion, together with Dr Tania Singer), says: "Even though there can be 'empathy fatigue', there cannot be 'compassion fatigue', since compassion is essentially a wholesome, positive state of mind, while empathy is only the tool that allows one to correctly perceive the state of mind of others."

People who care for others for a living, such as nurses, doctors and care workers, are susceptible to developing empathy fatigue.

So, are you suffering from empathy fatigue? Recognising your symptoms can help you take action before things get worse.

Signs of empathy fatigue can include:

- Depression
- Sudden outbursts of anger
- Feeling cynical or numb to what's happening around you
- Feeling isolated from family and friends

- Exhaustion
- Difficulty sleeping

You might want to take the Professional Quality of Life (ProQOL) test (details can be found in the Bibliography). This test identifies your levels of compassion satisfaction and empathy fatigue with your work. Read the questions as they relate to your workplace. There are things that you can do to minimise the risks to your mental health:

- Talk about and acknowledge your experiences with someone you trust, in enough detail to connect emotionally with them again.
- Brainstorm to find solutions that let you take action.
- Take care of yourself.

I worked in animal welfare and at a shelter for five years. I finally crumbled from empathy fatigue and walked off the job. Too late, I found a practice that could have enabled me to continue to enjoy the work I loved – mindfulness.

Unlocking the Benefits of Mindfulness

"Smile, breathe and go slowly." Thich Nhat Hanh

Learning mindfulness is proving extremely beneficial for people who suffer from empathy fatigue. Mindful and compassion practices increase empathy, compassion and coping skills among caregivers, and improve signs of depression, anxiety, stress and burnout. We become more aware of our thoughts, feelings and body sensations. The practices emphasise staying in the present moment, being non-judgemental, and striving towards an attitude of acceptance and kindness. The ultimate goal is to *respond* to situations instead of *reacting* to situations.

Mindfulness practice puts us in the present, in *this* moment. It's a self-directed practice for relaxing the body and calming the mind through focused, present-moment awareness. These practices help to move you from empathy and overwhelm to compassion, and feeling more positive emotions like care, love and wishing others well. Here are two of my favourite practices.

Mindful Walking meditation

"Walk as if you are kissing the Earth with your feet." Thich Nhat Hanh

This is referred to as a meditation, but you're walking slowly outside when you're doing it. No need to contemplate your navel!

Open the door and just start walking. Slowly. Look down to where you are placing your feet. Feel the weight as it rolls from your heel to your toes. Feel the support of the earth beneath your feet. Feel it pushing back. Notice how your weight shifts as you start to put pressure on your other foot. What are your arms doing? Are they comfortably at your sides, moving as you move? Are they out at your sides as you helicopter and try to keep your balance (if yes, slow your speed!). Be aware of your breath. Continue to walk mindfully for as long as you like.

Mindful Breathing

"Feelings come and go like clouds in a windy sky. Conscious breathing is my anchor." Thich Nhat Hanh

When you're feeling stressed, one great mindfulness exercise is to take slow deep breaths and just follow them. Feel the air entering your nostrils and reaching the back of your throat. Notice the rise and fall of your chest. Just be with yourself for a minute. It's amazing how quickly you can melt stress away just with your breath.

I share a guided three-minute breathing space meditation that you may like to try: visit TeachMindfulnessOnline.com/book.

If you wish to cultivate even more compassion, check out the loving-kindness meditation in our bonus audio tracks section – they have also been found to help people develop the skill of compassion and overcome empathy fatigue.

Remember:

- Limit your news intake to avoid being overwhelmed.
- Keep track of your feelings and state of mind, so you notice if you start to suffer from empathy fatigue and can take action.
- Take time throughout the day for simple mindfulness exercises to keep you feeling balanced.

About Michelle Alberigi McKenzie

Michelle is a certified Empathy Fatigue Educator and member of the Green Cross Academy of Traumatology. She is a certified intuitive life coach, a certified neuro-linguistic programming practitioner, a reiki master/teacher, and a mindfulness instructor. Michelle lives in the beautiful Sierra Nevada Foothills in California with her husband, dogs and cats.

www.MyPurposePath.com

Appendix

Audio Tracks

To listen to the free guided meditations and exercises that come with this book, visit: TeachMindfulnessOnline.com/book

Introduction: How to Use Mindfulness in Challenging Times by Shamash Alidina – *Inner advisor reflection*

Part 1 – Meeting Challenges with Mindfulness

Chapter 2: Staying Mindful in Isolation by Terry McCoy – *Antidote to isolation*

Chapter 4: Mindfulness for Anxiety by Caitriona Horan – *Mindful pause* and *Body scan*

Chapter 5: Managing Sleep in Challenging Times by Jane Bozier – *Mindful breathing*

Chapter 6: Mindfulness in the Presence of Traumatic Memories by Amy Malloy – *Coherent breathing*

Chapter 7: Being Mindful with Grief by Linda Shalloe – *Breathing in comfort meditation* and *'Hello Grief' poem*

Chapter 8: A Mindful Approach to Managing Your Media Consumption by Annemarie Wiegand – *Mindful media consumption meditation**

Part 2 – Practising Self-care, compassion and kindness

Chapter 9: Mindful Yoga by Jamila Knopp – *Alternate nostril breathing* and *Mindful yoga with body scan*

Chapter 11: Showing Ourselves Compassion by Stephanie Sackerman – *Self-compassion meditation*

Chapter 12: Growing Gratitude by Laura Goren – *Grounding gratitude meditation* and *Gratitude meditation*

Chapter 14: Micro-mindfulness Moments: Mindful Cleaning by Cheryl Green – *Washing hands mindfully meditation*

Chapter 15: Mindfulness for Finding Joy by Jennifer Gilroy – *Peace and freedom meditation*

Chapter 16: Connecting with Nature by Clare Snowdon – *Tree meditation* and *Natural object meditation*

Chapter 17: Mindful Movement in Nature by Lauretta Mazza – *Mindful movement in nature* and *More mindful movement*

Part 3 – Connecting Mindfully with Others

Chapter 18: Mindful Communication in Challenging Times by Calvin Niles – *Body scan meditation* and *Three-minute 'being present' meditation*

Chapter 19: Connecting with Others Online by Melissa Acuna-Dengo – *Connection meditation*

Chapter 20: Mindful Ways to Work from Home by Yvonne Cookson – *Guided image meditation for mental control for working from home*

Chapter 22: Mindful Ways through Conflict by Tosh Brittan – *Mindful ways through conflict meditation*

Chapter 23: Parenting Mindfully through Challenges by Crysal Olds – *A path to acceptance* and *Responding with compassion*

Chapter 24: Mindful Co-Parenting and Single Parenting by Elspeth Lewis – *A self-compassionate meditation for challenging times* and *Compassionate pause*

Chapter 25: Mindfulness for Helping Professionals by Karen Whitehead – *Checking in with yourself* and *Three-minute gratitude meditation for helping professionals*

Chapter 26: Mindfulness for Empathy Fatigue by Michelle Alberigi McKenzie – *Three-minute breathing space meditation*

Bonus Tracks

When you visit TeachMindfulnessOnline.com/book, you will also be able to access bonus tracks by other teachers in our community. Here is a list of some of them.

John Danias – *Mindfulness tips* and *Active meditation*
Deepanjali Sapotka – *Three-minute meditation* and *Ten-minute awareness meditation*
Robyn Zagoren – *Gratitude meditation*
Shamash Alidina – *Loving-Kindness meditation*

*Guided Meditation Music Credits: 'The Things That Keep Us Here' by Scott Buckley https://soundcloud.com/scottbuckley. Music promoted by https://www.free-stock-music.com. Attribution 4.0 International (CC BY 4.0)
https://creativecommons.org/licenses/by/4.0/

Bibliography

Chapter 1: Finding Calm in the Chaos
Bradt, S. (2010) Wandering mind not a happy mind. The Harvard Gazette. Available at:
https://news.harvard.edu/gazette/story/2010/11/wandering-mind-not-a-happy-mind/

Killingsworth, M. (2011) Want to be happier? Stay in the moment. TEDxCambridge. Available at:
https://www.ted.com/talks/matt_killingsworth_want_to_be_happier_stay_in_the_moment?language=en

Life change index stress test. Available at:
https://www.dartmouth.edu/eap/library/lifechangestresstest.pdf

McGonigal, K. (2013) How to make stress your friend. TEDGlobal. Available at:
https://www.ted.com/talks/kelly_mcgonigal_how_to_make_stress_your_friend

Track your happiness app: https://www.trackyourhappiness.org/

Chapter 3: Finding Ways to Cope with Stress
Davis, M., Eshelman, E.R. & McKay, M. (2008) *The Relaxation & Stress Reduction Workbook (6th ed.)*. Oakland, CA: New Harbinger Publications.

Selye, H. (1987) *Stress without Distress*. London: Corgi.

Chapter 4: Mindfulness for Anxiety

Alidina, S. (2015) *The Mindful Way Through Stress: The Proven 8-week Path to Health, Happiness, and Well-Being*. London: The Guilford Press.

Gilbert, P. (ed.) (2005) *Compassion: Conceptualisations, Research and Use in Psychotherapy*. London: Routledge.

Gilbert, P. (2013) *The Compassionate Mind*. London: Robinson.

Chapter 5: Managing Sleep in Challenging Times

Eugene, A. & Masiak, J. (2015) The neuroprotective aspects of sleep. *MEDtube Science*, 3(1), pp. 35–40.

Littlehales, N. (2016) *Sleep*. Milton Keynes: Penguin.

NHS (2019) How to get to sleep. Available at: https://www.nhs.uk/live-well/sleep-and-tiredness/how-to-get-to-sleep/

Chapter 6: Mindfulness in the Presence of Traumatic Memories

Harari, Y.N. (2015) *Sapiens: A Brief History of Humankind*. New York: Harper Perennial.

Porges, S.W. (2001) The polyvagal theory: Phylogenetic substrates of a social nervous system. *International Journal of Psychophysiology*, 42(2), pp. 123–146.

Treleaven, D.A. (2018) *Trauma-Sensitive Mindfulness: Practices for Safe and Transformative Healing.* New York: W.W. Norton & Co.

van der Kolk, B.A. (1994) The body keeps the score: Memory and the evolving psychobiology of posttraumatic stress. *Harvard Review of Psychiatry*, 1(5), pp. 253–65.

Chapter 7: Being Mindful with Grief

Kübler-Ross, E. & Kessler, D. (2005) *On Grief and Grieving: Finding the Meaning of Grief Through the Five Stages of Loss.* New York: Simon and Schuster.

Chapter 8: A Mindful Approach to Managing Your Media Consumption

AsapSCIENCE (not dated) 5 ways social media is changing your brain right now. TED-Ed. Available at: https://ed.ted.com/best_of_web/qQzsdX2Y

Charyk, C. (not dated) The mental trick you can use to get through any stressful situation. The Muse. Available at: https://www.themuse.com/advice/the-mental-trick-you-can-use-to-get-through-any-stressful-situation

Haynes, T. (2018) Dopamine, smartphones & you: A battle for your time. Harvard University. Available at: http://sitn.hms.harvard.edu/flash/2018/dopamine-smartphones-battle-time/

Statista (23 March 2020) Media Use – Statistics & Facts. Available at: https://www.statista.com/topics/1536/media-use/

Chapter 11: Showing Ourselves Compassion

Brach, T. (17 Jan 2020) Practice the RAIN meditation with Tara Brach. Available at: www.mindful.org/investigate-anxiety-with-tara-brachs-rain-practice/.

Neff, K. (2011) *Self Compassion: Stop Beating Yourself Up and Leave Insecurity Behind*. London: William Morris.

Neff, K. & Germer, C. (29 January 2019) The transformative effects of mindful self-compassion. Mindful. Available at: www.mindful.org/the-transformative-effects-of-mindful-self-compassion/

Chapter 12: Growing Gratitude
Emmons, R.A. & McCullough, M.E. (2003) Counting blessings versus burdens: An experimental investigation of gratitude and subjective well-being in daily life. *Journal of Personality and Social Psychology*, 84(2), pp. 377–389.

Lebya, E. (2016) Thanking others is actually good for you, research confirms. Psychology Today. Available at: https://www.psychologytoday.com/us/blog/joyful-parenting/201605/thanking-others-is-actually-good-you-research-confirms

Chapter 13: The Power of Being Kind to Others
Hamilton, D. (2019) *The Little Book of Kindness: Connect with Others, Be Happier, Transform Your Life*. London: Hachette.

Life Vest Inside: www.lifevestinside.com

Chapter 16: Connecting with Nature
Lowry C.A., et al. (2007) Identification of an immune-responsive mesolimbocortical serotonergic system: Potential role

in regulation of emotional behavior. *Neuroscience*, 146(2–5), pp. 756–772.

Chapter 22: Mindful Ways through Conflict
Alidina, S. (blog) *Kindfulness* by Ajahn Brahm: Book review and summary. Available at: https://www.shamashalidina.com/blog/kindfulness-by-ajahn-brahm-book-review-and-summary

Brown, B. (2011) The power of vulnerability. Available at: https://www.youtube.com/watch?v=iCvmsMzlF7o

PESI Inc. (2019) HALT: A mindful check in. Available at: https://www.youtube.com/watch?v=6YG4ujeNrO8

Yaribeygi, H., et al (2017) The impact of stress on body function: A review. *EXCLI Journal*, 16, pp. 1057–1072.

Chapter 23: Parenting Mindfully through Challenges
Faber, A. & Mazlish, E. (2013) *How to Be the Parent You Always Wanted to Be*. New York: Scribner.

Mead, E. (2020) 6 scales to measure coping and the brief cope inventory. Positive Psychology. Available at: https://positivepsychology.com/coping-scales-brief-cope-inventory/

Rexrode, K.R., Petersen, S. & O'Toole, S. (2008) The Ways of Coping Scale: A reliability generalization study. *Educational and Psychological Measurement*, 68(2), pp. 262–280.

Chapter 24: Mindful Co-parenting and Single Parenting
Segal, Z., Williams, M. & Teasdale, J. (2018) *Mindfulness-Based Cognitive Therapy for Depression (2nd ed.)*. London: Guilford Press.

Chapter 26: Mindfulness for Empathy Fatigue
Klimecki, O. & Singer, T. (2012) Empathic distress fatigue rather than compassion fatigue? Integrating findings from empathy research in psychology and social neuroscience. In: B. Oakley, A. Knafo, G. Madhavan, & D.S. Wilson (eds.), *Pathological Altruism*. New York: Oxford University Press, pp. 368–383.

Professional Quality of Life scale. Available at: https://proqol.org/uploads/ProQOL_5_English_Self-Score.pdf

Ricard, M. (2009) Empathy and the cultivation of compassion. Available at: https://www.matthieuricard.org/en/blog/posts/empathy-and-the-cultivation-of-compassion

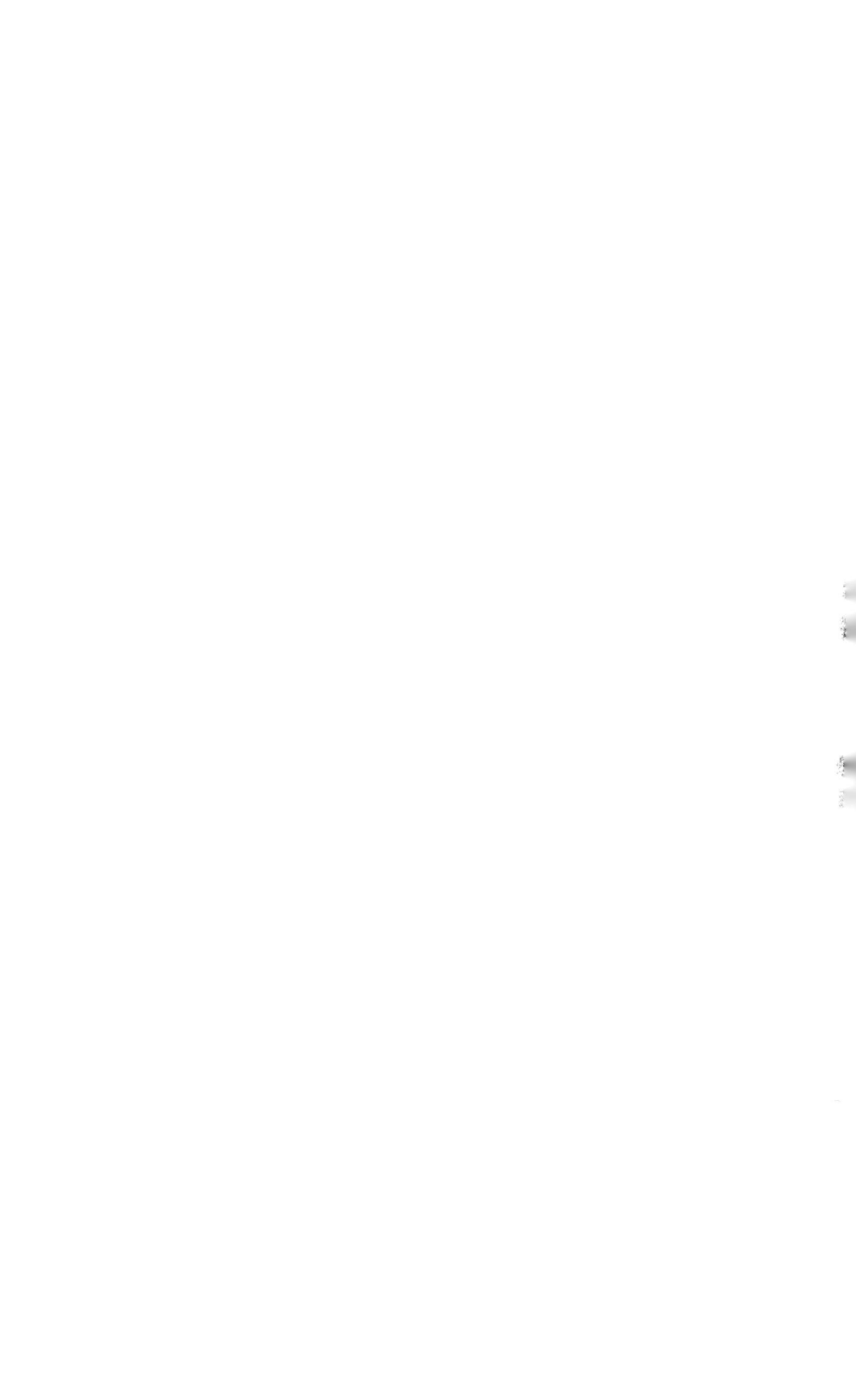

Printed in Poland
by Amazon Fulfillment
Poland Sp. z o.o., Wrocław